CW01020637

Hernia

Receive the Treatment to Cure Your Hiatus Hernia

(The Natural Solution to Hiatal Hernias So You Can Get Your Health Back)

Dennis Feliz

Published By **Simon Dough**

Dennis Feliz

Hernia: Receive the Treatment to Cure Your Hiatus Hernia (The Natural Solution to Hiatal Hernias So You Can Get Your Health Back)

ISBN 978-1-77485-869-1

No part of this guidebook shall be reproduced in any form without permission in writing from the publisher except in the case of brief quotations embodied in critical articles or reviews.

Legal & Disclaimer

The information contained in this ebook is not designed to replace or take the place of any form of medicine or professional medical advice. The information in this ebook has been provided for educational & entertainment purposes only.

The information contained in this book has been compiled from sources deemed reliable, and it is accurate to the best of the Author's knowledge; however, the Author cannot guarantee its accuracy and validity and cannot be held liable for any errors or omissions. Changes are periodically made to this book. You must consult your doctor or get professional medical advice before using any of the suggested remedies, techniques, or information in this book.

Upon using the information contained in this book, you agree to hold harmless the Author from and against any damages,

TABLE OF CONTENTS

Introduction

What exactly is Hiatus Hernia?

The description of hiatus hernia reads the displacement of a part of stomach through the diaphragm opening where the oesophagus travels between the chest and abdomen cavity.' In other words an area of the wall that is higher up the stomach extends through the diaphragm in the area that the gullet is able to pass between the chest and the abdominal cavity.

The diaphragm, or diaphragm, is a huge dome-shaped muscle that divides an abdominal space from the chest. This is the part of muscle that is concerned with breathing. It is supported by intercostal muscle (those in between the ribs) when you are working out. There are specific openings in it to permit the flow of blood vessels (the aorta as well as the Vena Cava) and also for the alimentary canal (the the oesophagus). The oesophageal opening (hiatus) that is of concern since

this is the place in which the hernia is formed and the opening in the oesophageal lining splits and grows larger and allows a portion of the stomach's wall to protrude out of.
Diaphragm when seen from below.
Hernias like this become more common as you age and it is estimated that around half of the population over 60 is affected by hiatus hernia but often without any symptoms. A barium X-ray is needed to determine the exact cause, however the diagnosis is determined by the identification of different signs and locations of tenderness and sensitivity. Hiatus hernia can be identified by pain in a variety of regions. The most common are between the sternum (breast bone) at the nipple level and, lower, behind the xiphoid artery at the top of the bone which is mostly cartilage (gristle). Other places of pain could be found on the left chest , and can be misinterpreted as angina. It can also be found near the base of the throat, or on the lower ribs

on the right; and, most often, through the back of that right shoulder blade.

Two different locations of pain

Hiccups may be due in the irritation caused by the phrenic nervous system if the hernia is large one. It is more painful when you bend in a tense manner, and also when lying down. "Heartburn" is the typical explanation for the pain and it is usually worse after eating. It is typically an overwhelming feeling of fullness and an increased amount of flatulence can be felt. Infrequently, nausea can be mentioned, and vomiting with projectiles can be seen in the most severe instances. As you'll see from the next pages the holistic method of healing will require time and dedication and dedication. However, the techniques of treatment are straightforward and safe.

The use of repressive therapy aimed to relieve symptoms primarily makes the condition worse. In this instance, the patient might feel more relaxed, however there is nothing being done to address the cause and the majority of drugs cause negative side effects of some type. Additionally the body must manage the drug while being in a weak or ill in a state of depletion. This is a way to increase the loss of vitality and weakens the body.

However, with natural remedies and a brief period of time patients experience feelings of relaxation and a boost in energy when there's still plenty to be done, and some of the symptoms could remain. The feeling of 'rightness' in the regimen, which provides the motivation to keep going. A lot of patients have told us that they didn't realize how much they were feeling after they'd tried the natural method of healing.

A holistic view is an way of living that is not only aimed at the treatment of ailments. If you follow this method and then implementing it, with a few modifications in the near future, many health issues can be avoided. I sincerely wish that you are motivated to alter your style of living, not only to treat your hiatus hernia, but also to improve your general health.

The natural healing process is slow. It is important to keep in mind that the problem is not a sudden occurrence - months or even years of postural and dietetic issues have contributed in the development of hiatus hernia. so it is reasonable that it may require several weeks changing to a healing situation, and another time in order to determine the pattern.

Chapter 1: The Causes Of Hiatus Hernia

In the naturopathic community, there is certain that this mechanical issue that is associated with hiatus hernias is due to the factors of modern western civilization such as obesity, sedentary work smoking, poor diet, shallow breathing, restrictive clothing, and emotional and mental tension.

Sedentary Occupations

If you don't engage in sensible - or regular physical activity, the body is predisposed to a variety of illnesses because cell activity decreases. That means the removal of waste is slower and not complete. The absorption of nutrients is slow, and metabolic rate is lower rate. This causes excessive accumulation of toxic matter within the body and the functional quality of being decreased.

It's not a good option to compensate for a sitting job with intense exercise on weekends. A lot of stress and strain is then imposed on a body that is not prepared and ill-suited for vigorous exercise. A steady, gradual training program is the ideal approach however if this isn't feasible, more gentle exercises, like swimming or walking without competition, are a good addition to the routine of the week. Dependence on automobiles and a inactivity at work are the cause of various mechanical problems in the body, which include varicose veins, spinal issues constipation, and the like however, they are also caused by a poor diet background.

Overweight

This can be due to eating too much eating, whether it's nibbling in between meals, eating excessively at meals or a combination of both. The larger meals pose the greatest threat to the health condition that we're discussing, as they raise the pressure on the diaphragm as a result of the massively enlarged and heavy stomach. However, excess weight is stressful and exhausting for the body. It causes a decrease in cell activity, decreased metabolic rate and a general "below the average' feeling. The fat (fatty) tissue can also compress the abdominal organs and diaphragm from the outside, preventing motion and the proper functioning of the organs and can cause constipation, that can exacerbate the toxic state.

Smoking and shallow breathing

Smoking cigarettes poses a threat to every condition. It's known the fact that lung cancer can be the result of smoking. But , besides this, the health of the whole is reduced due to the lack of air that circulates in the lungs and , consequently, in the bloodstream. The bloodstream, consequently is unable to deliver enough oxygen to tissues, or absorb the carbon dioxide that they release. Vitamin B's absorption is reduced and consequently the nervous system becomes more vulnerable. This causes a vicious cycle because smoking cigarettes is believed to stabilize the nerves. When a lack of exercise occurs with the consumption of unhealthy refined, over-processed and rich food It is clear that all the systems that are interconnected placed at risk and are prevented from producing any kind of well-being or wholeness.

It could be the result of smoking cigarettes, or could be caused by tight clothing or tension from everyday pressures and anxieties. The cause of shallow breathing is that the diaphragm muscles are held tight and only the chest moves when exhaling and inhaling. Because of a the absence of or infrequent use, the muscles are less toned and makes the diaphragm more susceptible to herniation. In addition the fact that breathing shallowly does not sufficiently aerate the lungs. This could results in less toxic elimination and lower absorption of. oxygen. A thorough exchange of gases in the lungs is vital to maintain good health.

It is easy to understand that breathing shallowly and smoking can lead to a variety of disorders, including digestive, circulatory, respiratory and nervous.

Impoverished Diet

There are a myriad of unwholesome ingredients that are used in products that fall under the label of food nowadays: for example the refined white flour that is found in many breads, cakes, biscuits and cakes as well as preservatives found in meats like salamis, sausages, and delicatessen chemical enhancers, chemicals and flavorings that are added to squashes and ice cream as well as refined sugars and syrups, and the excessive amount of salt found in a variety of packets and easy-cook items like instant mashed potatoes custard powders, convenience food items.

All of these should be avoided as the consumption of refined and devitalized food items results in less oxygen entering your body, than necessary. A lesser amount of minerals and vitamins are available to help balance and stimulate the proper nutrition. In the meantime, there is inadequate fibre available to enhance the peristaltic activity of the colon, and to maintain its health. In the end, every body tissue functions in a way that is not at their maximum potential. In fact, they function at lower than their normal capacity. The muscle tone decreases, and muscles become less resilient, and connective as well as fibrous tissues suffer from inadequate nutrition, and consequently is more susceptible to deterioration and atrophy. Additionally, the mucous membranes are thinner and more susceptible to irritation. It is therefore not surprising that the mucous membranes break down.

Drinks too can cause harm. Coffee and tea both cause irritation to the nervous system as well as the digestive tract and create acidic wastes that slow elimination. Squashes, coffee and alcohol all impact the mucous lining in the stomach. If these drinks are consumed in conjunction with meals or after when they are consumed, the weight of the stomach contents is increased which causes the stomach to stretch. This unwise combination also stimulates fermentation and creates gas which causes the stomach to expand. the stomach can be increased and causes pressure on the diaphragm and Oesophageal opening. This is a significant factor in exacerbating the possibility of hernias.

"We are what we consume It is the responsibility of every person to have a balanced diet that provides your body with the essential raw materials needed for proper functioning. This way, health is preserved and illness is prevented. A healthy diet should consist of at minimum fifty per 100 percent fruits and vegetables and at minimum, half of it is uncooked. Other food categories like carbohydrates as well as proteins and fats should comprise the remaining 50 percent. If we consume and drink well functionally, the quality of every system of the body is improved. In turn, we can think more clearly and behave with greater precision and awareness.

In a number of instances of hiatus hernia,, it is known that air-swallowing may be a cause that can aggravate the condition because it expands the stomach. This is typically the case when the stomach is filled through food. One method to avoid this is to to breathe out every time food is put in the mouth. Additionally, take your time eating, and eating the food slowly and thoroughly.

Tight-fitting clothing

A waist-length restriction can cause compression. This impacts the digestive system, circulatory and nervous systems especially the diaphragm as well as the respiratory system. The body's movement is limited and bodily functions are impaired. Women, for instance prefer wearing bras and girdles that are overlapping around the waist, forming an'spare tyre'. Although this could achieve their purpose, this type of clothes are detrimental to health and can be an extremely risk factor for the development of hiatus hernia, as it hinders the full range of motion that the diaphragm can make.

Emotional and Mental Tension

Mental and emotional stress and anxiety trigger the vagus nerve as well as the sympathetic nervous system. The most obvious part that is affected by this condition is the solar plexus , which is where the sensation of "butterflies is experienced when we are stressed. When we are anxious, the solar plexus gets tighter and the sensation experienced feels like a large lump. We all know the horrible feeling of sickness when we see an incident on the highway. Resentment, anger, jealousy and self-pity are all triggered by this precisely tuned "relay station' that is designed to increase the flow of adrenalin and increase heartbeat and blood flow. Other metabolic changes can include increased breathing that corresponds to a higher pulse as well as the slowing of digestive functions as well as the growth and repair processes. In the case of chronic anxiety, all of this happens, but less evidently, it is affecting function and limiting diaphragmatic motion that is essential for good health and prevention of hiatus hernia.

Chapter 2: Relaxation Of Hiatus Hernia

What can you do to manage this painful illness? It is obvious that you must restore the body in all its entirety; it is a daunting task, however when you take it slow, step-by-step with a steady, positive attitude the new routine isn't too difficult and, as your system of the body is relieved by the treatment, you will feel urge to continue. Before starting the actual procedure it is a good option to lift the top of the bed with bricks that are used can be placed the bed's legs or by pushing the mattress up by using a bolster that is very sturdy or a piece of wood, or the wedge shape of foam rubber. (More pillows can be utilized.) This can help stop the vomiting of food throughout the night and help relieve stomach acid and flatulence.

It is crucial to be able to breathe correctly and using diaphragm. Diaphragmatic breathing is actually simple, and the next routine should be highly recommended.

Figure 3 Diaphragmatic breathing

Relax on the floor with your knees bent, and feet close to your buttocks. As you relax your body. Put your hands gently on your abdomen (note that this isn't illustrated in the diagram, to prevent obscuring abdominal movement) and keep your focus to this region. Then breathe in slowly, gently pressing the abdomen upwards underneath your hands simultaneously until you are able to breathe out completely. is inhaled. Relax, breathe out through your mouth, making the sound of an audible sighing. let the abdominal wall receding (see illustration). The chest and shoulders should be relaxed throughout the exercise.

There may initially be a desire to "suck into' the abdomen to increase the chest size, as that is the way to be understood through deep breathing and certain ways of teaching stress breathing through the chest, as it is the primary aspect of breathing. The chest certainly plays an important role, however the the diaphragm enhances the effectiveness of the lungs, by using the lung's deeper tissue. A tempo-based exercise, or training to improve the lung's capacity, has an effect of massaging on the abdominal organs, thereby stimulating the body's function.

A truly complete breath starts with the diaphragm , and is followed by the intercostal muscles which help expand the lungs upwards, above and sides to sides. Take a full breath at least at least once. It is exhausting to breathe this in a manner for so long but it's beneficial when exercising. In the normal course of life breath is an automatic and when the diaphragm is not affected in a negative manner due to tension, anxiety or keeping the tummy in the interest of appearance, it will perform its job efficiently.

Return, and then back to the training. It's best to practice it early in the morning and the last first thing at night. Start with five or six "tummy" breaths and then increase it one breath per day until fifteen. Be at ease and don't use any the force. If there is any feeling of strain or a feeling of discomfort, it is because excessive effort has been applied; pushing hard at it is not helping the goal. Refresh yourself slowly after (especially following the morning workout) since deep breathing is usually associated with some sensation of excitement. It's normal, and it is caused by the acceleration of circulation, and then goes off in a couple of minutes. In the daytime, occasionally, attempt to perform the same breathing while sitting well supported in a chair, and then in walking and standing. Don't fret when it doesn't be working. The act of directing thoughts towards the diaphragm assists in promoting its work and it becomes easier with each session. This breathing technique can reduce pain, and should be practiced every time you experience an injury.

It is crucial to be able to unwind whenever you want to as, with the development and practice of this ability can stop mental and bodily tensions from growing into a level that causes physical symptoms. In the beginning lay on a firm surface (though it could initially be uncomfortable It is much harder to fool yourself, and it has more value than a cushioned couch or bed). A sleeping bag placed on the floor is ideal and, in summertime conditions, a rug laid on the lawn will be a dream - relaxation isn't possible in frigid conditions.

The key to relaxation is to become conscious of your physical body and mind in a constructive light. When you are aware, you have the ability to sense stress and tension immediately and to recognize that the build-up can't happen if the tension is relieved in the initial moment. To make the distinction between relaxation and tension more evident to the student it is necessary to perform a series movements of tensing and relaxing multiple joint and muscle groups is performed, starting by releasing the feet and progressing all the way to the head. This is done in sync with breathing. It is done by following this pattern:

1. Breathe in and then bend your feet to 90 degrees. Keep them for a few seconds and note the tightness within the muscles of the shins as well as the ankle joints. Breathe in a sigh and let go Do not try to do anything during this portion of the exercise just let go of the tension that is created by bending your feet upwards. Repeat this once.

2 Turn your focus up towards your knees. Breathe deeply as you press both knees to the ground, noticing the tightness in the muscles in the thigh. Breathe in to exhale and then let them go. Repeat.

3. Focus your attention on the buttocks. Breathe into as you contract (squeeze) the muscles. (Try not to squeeze any other part of your body. It is possible to notice yourself clenching your jaws or

hands to help the process, but this should be avoided.) Take note of the tension and let it release as you breathe out and then sigh. Repeat.

4. Think about your abdominal region (tummy). The muscles are pulled back as if they be able to touch your spine as you breathe into (the opposite of diaphragmatic breathing). Keep them for several seconds, taking note of the pain, then breathe out and relax the muscles. Repeat.

5 The hands are the next on the list. You need to clench your hands really tight and increase the grip as you breathe in . you will feel the blockage that tension can cause. Sigh out and then let go of your hands. It should bring an euphoria in the event that the grip was tight. Repeat.

6 Bend your elbows with a firm force and bring hands to shoulders, breathe in - breath out, then release like before. Repeat.

7. Next, while breathing in, pull the shoulder blades in a tight way and note the discomfort then let it go, breathing deeply. Repeat.

8 Now, the facial muscles will tighten. The muscles around the eyes, and frown. squeeze the jaw while breathing into. Release the jaw with a sigh. Repeat.

9 Complete this initial section by putting every 'tensing' and then stiffen your entire body. Then, 'fall into an 'assembly', to speak, before releasing and exhaling. Repeat.

It is a lot of effort to achieve this, but the ease of letting go of the tension is evident. Begin with three or four deep, slow diaphragmatic breathswhile in a state of sigh as you exhale. Start to quiet your mind by consciously imagining the most beautiful spot - a place unique to you - peaceful and deserted. Then you can imagine yourself in that place. Explore it with your mind's eye , and take in the beauty of it; feel you are part of the beautiful scene. Don't pay attention to your body, and open up to these beautiful surroundings. Think of yourself as a an integral part of this universe (which it is) and essential to the overall scheme of things. Reach a point where you are happy relaxed, peaceful, warm and sleepy, and then stay there for a couple of minutes (or for as long as you're able). The thoughts of your day will come into your head from time to at will; it is best to allow them to drift by without getting frustrated or pursuing them. After that, you can go back to your imagined beautiful spot. As time passes, your active mind will be calming and the thoughts that distract you will diminish and then cease however this could require several weeks of consistent practice. Once you're ready take a break from the wonderful location, return to your present moment, yawn and stretch out and "wake up'. Start slowly as sleeping can reduce metabolism and rushing up could cause a minor stress to the body.

In addition, if you're in the vicinity of a cell phone then either place it in cushions or get from the hook. You can see that the goal of this is to totally detached from the world for a time, and let your body and mind to recharge and rest. When you do it daily starting with ten minutes, moving to twenty minutes, and then working up to an hour or so the conscious mind as well as your subconscious mind will be trained . And, eventually, you'll discover that you're not so stressed about the world, that anxiety does not linger as long and that you're more calm. This method is extremely helpful in any situation where tension and anxiety are a factor.

Chapter 3: Diet

We are at the point at which preconceived notions need to be dismantled and new ideas embraced; therefore, it is essential to be open to adopting an entirely new perspective and explore the new ideas by keeping an open-minded mind.

Habits and addictions

Start, if you smoke to quit, by quitting or If you are able to do it to cut back, reduce it by four cigarettes every day slowly. While this may be difficult, you should keep in mind the fact that your entire body will gain once the withdrawal issues are resolved. Drink one cup (not cup) of substitute coffee as well as a cup of tea every daily. Other times, drink juices of vegetables or fruits and herbal teas like peppermint, camomile and lime or fennel, or drinks such as Barley Cup or a dandelion coffee. There are a variety of options that can be found at health food stores. While you're there be sure to keep track of your time for drinking and eating Take water half an hour prior to the meal or for two hours after. This aids digestion significantly and decreases the risk of heartburn. Drinking during meals increases the overall weight of the stomach, which slows the digestion process, as it dilutes the digestive juices, which in turn increases the chance of gas formation and fermentation that expands the stomach and creates pressure and, consequently, discomfort and discomfort.

Every meal should be smaller in size than normal eating on a smaller plate can help, and a complete mastication is crucial in order to break down food into small particlesand reduce the speed of consumption. An approximate estimate is approximately thirty-two to forty chews for every mouthful. Do not count every bite eaten. Take note of chewing more deeply and now and then, keep a record, to see how close the mark you reach. Naturally, it's going to depend on the kind of food consumed which is a further issue; in the end the diet will include more fruits and vegetables than in the past and less refined, soft and processed foods such as white bread and biscuits, cakes and sugar rice puddings and cooked vegetables. I have mentioned in the beginning that repetition can aid in highlighting that a healthy diet must comprise at least fifty percent fruits and vegetables and 50 per cent in total, of carbohydrates, protein and fat. It is a goal. It is not achievable in a hurry, but keeping these principles in your mind and striving to achieve them will aid the overall goal.

Raw Juices

If you suffer from hiatus hernia, it's crucial to incorporate juices from the raw source into your diet as quickly as you can.

But, the digestive tract may be sensitive at first so it is recommended that freshly prepared, raw carrot juice is consumed for at least half an hour prior to each meal, including breakfast. Even without a juice extractor, it is still possible to make in a very simple manner, and directions are provided, along with recipes and sample menus within this book. Carrot juice is a highly relaxing effect as it is a great source of calcium and vitamin A as well as an alkaline component which is a soothing ingredient for stomach. Be persistent with this, even though the flavor of carrot juice is quite bland. Be aware the fact that any juice, vegetables or fruits, should be slightly dilute because they tend to be concentrated. Make sure to add 1 tablespoon of water for every 120 milliliters of juice. either tap water or bottle water is suitable. Alternate the recipe later by mixing fresh apple juice and carrot, and using beetroot and apple juice or celery and beetroot however, these juices require a juicer that is properly designed. The canned varieties of fruit juice are very good however, they've had to be processed, which means that some oxygen and vitamins is lost. However, it's simple and easy method to get juices.

It is important to note that the juice of beetroots and beetroots when consumed in any amount can cause coloration of blood (pink) and the faeces (dark dark red). This is normal and is not an indication of illness.

Basic Principles of Healthy Eating

Consume only whole food items; which means only items that aren't been refined to remove their original goodness from them, which happens with white rice, white flour and the like.

Eat those foods that have not been contaminated with unnecessary/flavourings, colourings, 'improvers', preservatives, or heavy salt and sugar additives. Food additives like these needs been made clear on packaging or in tins as per law, therefore, read the label!

Fish and meat that are canned generally heavily salted or processed with preservatives, so you should be cautious of these products - as well as high-spiced and preserved delicatessen cuts of meat. A lot of cheeses contain salt, so make sure to look for brands that are low in sodium or varieties.

Consume a lot of fruits, salads and grains, seeds, nuts and pulses as well as all kinds of vegetables. Dried fruits are excellent, however, they can be a bit rattler concentrated therefore should be consumed in a balanced manner by fresh fruits as well as mineral water. Fish, meat, poultry eggs, cheese All proteins need to be balanced by plenty of vegetables in order to maintain an acceptable acid-alkali balance.

I've said before that any diet must comprise fifty percent fruits and vegetables, in order to counterbalance an acidity from the remaining fifty percent of food items which include carbohydrates, proteins , and/or fats.

The average diet gives too enough attention to protein. A daily intake of 115-170 grams is sufficient for those who is not engaged in strenuous, physical activity. There are many other sources of protein , including the fruits, seeds grains, pulses and grains.

A greater attention should be given to the balance of the diet to ensure that minerals, vitamins and fiber all play an important role. So, your body can get the maximum amount of the substances required to be healthy.

The enjoyment of food is crucial, and food items with attractive designs stimulate digestive juices and enhance the enjoyment of eating food and help digestion.

A relaxed and comfortable eating environment taking time to eat slowly, and chewing food properly, all have been discussed before but are the foundation of good digestion , and should be taken into consideration.

Your New Diet

It's a good idea to start the day in a healthy way by introducing something that is beneficial to the body. Instead of the standard cup of tea which can over-stimulate the nervous system and can cause irritation to the stomach's lining and raises acidity in the bloodstream Take a cup of herbal tea. They have a softer effect and stimulate the healing power that the body has. The tea helps digestion, eases flatulence, and improves the stomach's lining. Chamomile helps to calm nerves and can be great for colic. Hence, it is a great choice to drink to drink in the morning and, when taken together it will reap the advantages of both.

Make sure that hot drinks cool slightly before drinking. Temperature fluctuations in food as well as drinks, should be avoided. And just like food should be consumed slowly, drinks should also be consumed slowly.

Some people may be more appropriate to their specific personality and the environment of the house to make the adjustments slowly. Natural processes are slow and it's much wise to adjust your lifestyle gradually and in a consistent manner, than jump into a situation only to soon find that you are unable to keep it up. Additionally abrupt changes can trigger an allergic reaction in the body, possibly temporarily causing symptoms to worsen that could serve as an obstacle to continuing to eat.

Making a plan for use across the board is challenging since everyone is different. The recommended amounts in the plan is the upper limit. People with a large appetite might feel extremely hungry or feeling empty, so it is possible to increase the amount stated, typically with spoons (by between one and three times an example of the highest). Be careful and take the most minimal amount recommended if you can.

Week One

Make use of this week in the following ways:

1. Learn breathing and relaxation techniques.

2 Drink 120 milliliters of freshly-made carrot juice 30 minutes prior to each meal. Make sure that it is consumed.

3 Eat and drink at different time.

4. If you need to you must cut out (or lower) smoking.

5 Consume only the equivalent of one cup coffee and tea each day.

6 Start the day with a cup of peppermint or chamomile tea.

7 Eat smaller portions of food, and chew them thoroughly.

8 Increase the bed head's height by four to 10 centimeters and then gradually get into the feeling of the new routine.

Let the natural forces within the body take over and correct the imbalance that's been in place for a long time and eventually the eight elements will result in improvement. In fact, any of them will help small amount. (See the section on Hydrotherapy)

The next week will be adhering to a more strict plan designed to rid the body of harmful wastes and accelerating healing processes, while at the same time reducing discomfort and pain.

The diet is easy at first, with the natural whole foods, and a small amounts of mixtures to aid in digestion. As time goes on, more foods which are high in oxygen minerals, vitamins and oxygen are introduced to aid in healing and overall health. A balanced diet that is based on whole food, obviously, and, ideally, vegetarian, is recommended at the conclusion this course. The last phase, the one that deals with the hiatus hernia, is going to be the beginning of a completely new way of living that will not lead back to the previous unhealthy ways of life. This should be a lifestyle that is more energetic and more capacity to leisure and work and a life that is based on more expansive concepts and spiritual understanding and a lifestyle of good health.

Week Two

The most important food item for your week's meals is brown rice as it's a source of silica, a mineral that aids the body get rid of harmful substances and helps in promoting healing, particularly for digestive issues. Brown rice retains its bran that is natural, and is less brittle than wheat bran which means it provides more bulk to the body without causing irritation. Rice is primarily an agrarian food that is starchy, however it contains around 8 per cent protein and also some trace amounts in calcium, phosphorus as well as in addition, several B vitamins, including Niacin, thiamine and in lesser amounts the Riboflavin. These vitamins are beneficial for nourishing your nervous system which is well-known.

Three main dishes are rice-based. The rice is cooked, and it can make a huge difference in the event that enough rice can be cooked to last two days. Rinse 225g of rice through a sieve and then place it in 570ml of boiling water. To this, 1 teaspoon sunflower oil is added. (This assists in keeping the grains in a separate.) Let it simmer slowly until the water has been absorbed - around twenty to 25 minutes. Pour it into the container or basin with lid and then it's ready to put it in the refrigerator or in a cool area. The quantity recommended is very small, and deliberately however, should you really require more, a bit could be added.

Week Two Day One

7 a.m. The moment you awake the next day, try chamomile or peppermint tea.

8. a.m. 120 milliliters freshly prepared carrot juice.

8.30 a.m. 8.30 a.m. Breakfast 3 standard tablespoons of cooked rice and 3 tablespoons of stewed apples sweetened by honey (this could be warmed to your liking if you prefer).

10.30 a.m. Barley Cup.

12.30 p.m. Carrot juice.

1 p.m. Lunch 3 tablespoons rice with 1 tablespoon of freshly grated raw carrot. 1 tablespoon minced parsley. (This gives Vitamins A and C as well as as well as calcium as well as potassium.) A small

amount of the yeast extract, or even soya sauce may be added.

3. p.m. China tea or herb tea.

5 p.m. Carrot juice.

5.30 p.m. Dinner Three tablespoons rice, with

4 to 6 apricots or prunes that have been left to soak over night, and not cooked along with 2 tablespoons yogurt made from natural.

7.30 p.m. Barley Cup or herb tea followed, about an hour prior to bedtime by 4 5 fl 1 oz (120 milliliters) the juice of a red grape, with plenty of mineral water. It is a great beverage to sooth and relax, as well as a digestive also.

Sleep is likely to be comfortable with this method, because there won't be food left in the stomach at the time you go to bed; and if you drink the drink of the night half an hour prior to going bed, it will be in digestion. The diaphragmatic breathing can also be helpful in bringing you to sleep. (See the information about cold packs treatment)

Week Two Day Two

This is a repeat of the day before however, the amount of food may have to be adjusted by a small amount. It is essential that the bowels of the lower part be free of obstruction; and because the total volume of bulk that is consumed is lower than usual, there might be constipation for a short period of time. Apricots or prunes that you ate in the night before can keep this from occurring. If, however, this second day is not followed by a motion, there's the option of using an herbal laxative or a full dessert spoon of black treacle, which is half a tumbler of hot or warm water.

Week Two Day Three

This is a diet that is progressive and the intention, throughout it, will be to boost the quantity of raw food consumed because they promote healing and increase the quality of health in general. If you combine whole grains, vegetable and grain proteins as well as unsaturated oils as well as natural sugars an ideal equilibrium is created. There are many different individuals, of course and, when offering general advice, it's impossible to address specific demands. If a person thinks they require individual assistance should seek out an expert Naturopath.

7. a.m. herbal tea just like before.

8. a.m. A fresh cup of carrot juice.

8.30 a.m. breakfast 3-4 tablespoons of rice cooked with 6 apricots or prunes, 2 tablespoons of natural yogurt as well as 1 teaspoon of almonds that have been ground.

10.30 a.m. Barley Cup or similar.

12.30 p.m. Juice of fresh carrots.

1 p.m. Lunch: 3-4 tablespoons of cooked brown rice, 1 tablespoon chopped raw carrots, one teaspoon chopped chopped parsley. One teaspoon sunflower seeds 6-8 sprigs of watercress chopped and mixed in the rice along with 2 or 1 tablespoons of natural yogurt, and a tiny amount, such as a teaspoon of extract yeast.

3.30 p.m. China -tea or herbal tea.

5.30 p.m. Carrot juice.

6.00 p.m. Dinner brown rice, like before, tossed with one raw apple grated including skin and Pips, soaked prunes or Apricots, 1 tablespoon ground almonds, and 2 tablespoons of yogurt made from natural sources (with some honey, if needed).

8.30 p.m. Barley cup or tea with peppermint.

9.30/10 p.m. Grape juice red like before.

Week Two Day Four

This is a repeat that occurred on Day Three. As we are now assuming that it will be the 2nd week of your illness, there is a noticeable decrease in symptoms is expected and some energy is accessible. The nervous system will feel more calm. Every day, the diet is going to become more interesting.

Week Two Day Five

The same routine starting with the breakfast drink and the carrot juice.

Breakfast The ideal breakfast is a raw apple grated with 4 to 6 Apricots or prunes, 1 tablespoon of almonds ground 2 tablespoons of organic yogurt and a banana that is ripe.

In the middle of morning: Barley Cup or dandelion coffee

Apple juice.

Before lunch: Tomato juice.

Lunch: 115 grams cottage cheese, in the mix is 1 tablespoon of mint chopped one grated carrot 1 teaspoon sunflower seeds, one dessert spoon of raisins one tomato (scalded and removed from the skin) 1 teaspoon cider vinegar, and some watercress sprigs.

Mid-afternoon: Herbal China tea or juice from bottled fruit (apple or pineapple).

Prior to dinner After dinner, drink tomato juice or carrot juice.

Evening meal: 2 potatoes (small), steamed. With their skins still on, 2 small carrots (small) 2 8 oz (55 grams) in frozen peas one teaspoon polyunsaturated margarine 1 tablespoon of extract from yeast.

Routine prior to completing the evening.

Week Two Day Six

Repetition Day Five.

Week Two Day Seven

Follow the same routine between meals.

Breakfast: Muesli: Overnight, soak 2 tablespoons of flaked oats , or wheat for 4 cups of water. The next morning, add 1 raw apple grated one dessert spoon of raisins and 8 chop almonds and 1 teaspoon the powdered milk (or 2 teaspoons of yogurt) and 1 teaspoon of honey. Take this seriously and chew it thoroughly.

Lunch lunch: 2 or 3 lettuce leaves and 4 or 5 sprigs watercress, 1 skinned tomato, grated raw carrot 1 small grated raw beetroot and sunflower seeds. 1/2 an apple cut or chunked, 115 grams cottage cheese 2 teaspoons of cider vinegar sprinkled on 2 or 3 steamed potatoes with skins left on.

Evening meal: Steamed vegetables The heart of the cabbage (if not too large) 2 carrots, one small onion, either a green or red pepper, cut into cabbage, then steamed and grated 55 g Cheshire cheese sprinkled on top. (Note that peppers are rich in vitamin C, and they retain much of it in the cooking process.)

This is the end of your second week. The next step is to assess yourself. What are your results in your assessment? Are you satisfied with the progress you've made? Do you feel hungry after eating? If yes, it will disappear as your stomach returns to its normal size. If your meals become more extensive, do you have any pain or flatulence? Flatulence can last for a few weeks but it will be less frequent and in volume. Are you feeling more relaxed and positive? Write down what is left to be accomplished you are happy and satisfied with your accomplishments to date.

Week Three

Many changes will be implemented in your diet during this time, and will progress to a normal, reformed diet after the 4th week. The changes could be too swift for some people, and a small recrudescence could be observed. If this happens you should go back to the stage that brought you the most satisfaction for a few days, and then attempt to progress once more. There is no point in insisting on progress if it will have negative effects.

Day One of Week Three

The first thing to do is wake up 2 teaspoons cider vinegar, and a teaspoon of sugar in hot water.

Before breakfast: 120ml of apple juice in a bottle.

Breakfast: Muesli with prunes and yogurt.

11 a.m. Coffee-type drink.

After lunch: Vegetable juice Choose from carrots beetroot, celery, beetroot tomatoor combination of two.

Do not exceed 120 milliliters as you normally would.

Lunch Salad: Keep portions of salads to a minimum. Make use of a slice of pepper and watercress, lettuce beetroot, carrots, tomatoes, sunflower seeds mint and cottage cheese. To meet the requirement for starch, you can have one slice of 100 % wholewheat bread and margarine with polyunsaturated. For dessert, try an apple.

4. p.m. China or herb tea, as previously.

Prior to dinner Before dinner: Grapefruit juice.

Dinner: poached eggs on mashed carrots with a green vegetables in season, and potatoes wrapped in skin. Dessert: Apple or pear.

After 2 hours: A coffee drink is recommended if you are in need.

Prior to bedtime: the standard grape juice.

Week Three Day Two

The first thing to do: When you wake up in the morning, use the cider vinegar like before.

Prior to breakfast Drinking apple juice before breakfast.

Breakfast The perfect breakfast is a banana, eight dates, almonds An apple and yogurt, or 120ml untreated milk.

11 a.m. Grapefruit juice.

Prior to lunch After lunch: Mineral water.

Lunch: Salad like before, but with 55 grams of milled nuts (not peanuts) to provide protein, and potatoes as starch.

To eat dessert, a piece of apple.

4 p.m. The tea will be served as usual.

Before dinner Before dinner: Grapefruit juice.

Evening dinner: Grilled whitefish Cod, haddock or plaice fillet. peas and carrots.

For dessert, try grapes or pear.

You can follow this up with the standard nighttime beverage.

Week Three Day Three

The first thing to do: early drinks like prior to.

Breakfast Eggs boiled one slice of 100 percent wholemeal bread, and margarine that is polyunsaturated. Two or three apples.

Mid-morning: Grapefruit juice.

Prior to lunch After lunch: Mineral water.

Lunch: Salad: Try different ingredients, e.g. cucumber or celery 55 grams Cheddar cheese, one or two potatoes.

To serve as dessert, soak or soaked apricots, prunes or apricots.

4 p.m. The usual tea.

Prior to dinner After dinner, drink a glass of pineapple juice.

Evening dinner: Millet and Tomato Savoury with carrots and other green vegetables. Dessert: Grapes or an apple.

For the remainder of the week To complete the week, you must repeat the three days previously listed, and then repeat Day One over and over. If the diet plan has been followed and you have made progress, then the next week may begin with confidence.

Week Four

Monday

First , choose among cider vinegars juices from fruits and herbal tea.

Prior to breakfast Before breakfast: Mineral water.

breakfast: natural yogurt, honey, apple, between 8 and 12 grapes, and a pear. This yogurt is consumed in its entirety or is made into a fruit salad with the yogurt drizzled over.

Mid-morning Drinks of yeast extract that are savoury dilute with milk and water carrot juice or tea.

Before lunch: Pineapple juice.

LunchSalad lettuce tomatoes (skinned) chopped carrot, beetroot and grated some sliced pepper sprouted seeds of alfalfa, two slices of 100 percent whole wheat bread, and unsweetened butter. A hard-boiled egg. Make use of apple cider vinegar, sunflower oil and sunflower to make a salad dressings or, alternatively yogurt.

Fresh fruit as dessert.

The mid-afternoon hours: China tea.

Prior to dinner Before dinner: Pineapple juice.

Dinner The first course is half an avocado, drizzled with vinaigrette dressing.

The second course Cauliflower vegetables, courgettes, and carrots (in season) 55 g grated Cheddar cheese to sprinkle on the vegetables. Fresh fruit is next.

Evening drinks before.

Tuesday

Note: Between breakfast or lunch, as well as dinner beverages should be arranged in the same way as previously.

Breakfast Apricots and prunes that have been soaked 1 teaspoon of sunflower seeds. 1 dessert spoon of almonds that have been ground and natural yogurt.

Lunch Salad: Watercress, beetroot, celery and orange.

Dressing Mixture: Yogurt and chopped Mint.

Try cottage cheese and potatoes to make this. Take as much as like and are at ease with. Fresh fruits to follow.

Dinner The first course is avocado and vinaigrette salad dressing.

Second course: Omelette of mushrooms Peas, runner beans or peas and carrots.

Desserts: Apple Crumble or fruit cake.
Wednesday
(Keep your regular routine of drinking.)
Breakfast An egg boiled two slices of 100 percent wholemeal bread, margarine that is polyunsaturated, as well as an apple.

Lunch lunch: Grated carrot, grated apple raw beetroot grated 1 tablespoon of sunflower seeds 1 teaspoon of chopped parsley, 115 grams of cottage cheese 2 breads with rye crisps as well as polyunsaturated margarine.

French dressing. A fresh banana and yogurt are the next ingredients.

Dinner The first course is half an orange. The second dish: Cheesy Soya Mix, green vegetables (e.g. cabbage) Leeks, carrots, and carrots (in the season) as well as onions.

Dessert Apricots and prunes soaked with yogurt made of goat's milk.

Thursday
Breakfast: Home-made Muesli.

Lunch Salad: Mixed: Lettuce watercress, tomatoes, lettuce (skinned) and 1 small raw courgette, chopped, grated carrot several raisins and a slice of onion as well as mint and yogurt dressing. Slice of 100% percent whole wheat bread, butter, as well as 1 tablespoon of almonds ground.

Evening meal: First course: Tomato salad. Second course The second course is The third course is an Egg and Cheese Bake and peas, or runners beans and carrots and courgettes.

Dessert: Fresh fruit.

Friday

Breakfast Fruits: Fresh grapes, an orange or apple, and a few nuts and dates preferred hazelnuts or almonds.

Lunch Salad: Sprouted Alfalfa seeds coleslaw or fresh cabbage and carrots and some onion as well as vinaigrette salad dressing. Two or three potatoes. Prunings that have been soaked to follow.

Dinner The first course is half of a grapefruit. The second dish: Stuffed Pepper, carrots and green vegetables (in season).

Desserts: Apples baked filled with dates or raisins.

Saturday

Breakfast: Sliced and fruit and raisins, sunflower seeds as well as natural yogurt.

Lunch Salad: Mixed cooked beetroot, chopped and diced apple, celery and walnuts, tossed with vinaigrette dressing. Two rye crispbreads served with cottage cheese.

Fresh fruit, such as grapes and peaches (in season).

Evening meal: First course: Tomato salad. The second course is Chestnut Pudding (page 94) served with green vegetables including carrots, peas, and carrots.

Dessert: Fresh fruit salad.

Sunday

Breakfast: Scrambled eggs with toast with an apple.

Lunch First course: Half of a grapefruit.

The second course Cauliflower vegetables, cheese and courgettes.

Dessert Baked apples.

Evening dinner: Fresh fruit A pear or orange, grapes, apricots, and raisins.

The weeks of Weeks 5 and 6

The two-week menus will assist you in following the previous regimen and will provide a framework to help you plan for the future.

The drinks you drink the first thing in the morning are not listed in any particular order to help you remember it is possible to pick from:

Cider vinegar, hot water and honey

Lemon juice squeezed hot water, honey, and hot water,

Herbal teas of your choice: Chamomile, peppermint, etc.,

Fruit juices - orange, apple, pineapple, etc.

Similar to the drink you have before bed. Pick from:

Slippery Elm Food,

Red grape juice (red) hot or cold
Vecon (with the addition of milk).
Be aware that drinks are to be 1'2 tumbler in amount, except for the lastly, if more than double the amount is consumed and drunk in a continuous manner.

Monday

Breakfast: Baked prunes, and yogurt made from natural sources.

Mid-morning: Con with a some milk.

Lunch Salad: grated carrots and watercress, 1/2 apple and tomato (scalded as well as skinned) with sunflower seeds, and raisins. Dressing cider vinegar, sunflower oil. Baked jacket potatoes and some butter, 2 tablespoons of ground almonds.

Mid-afternoon The best herbal Tea or Rosehip Peppermint and Chamomile.

Prior to dinner Before dinner: Pineapple juice.

Evening meal: Whole wheat macaroni and homemade tomato sauce cooked broccoli and steamed carrots (or like it). Baked apple with dates.

Tuesday

Breakfast: Apples sliced raw and Muesli.

In the middle of the morning: Barley Cup (or similar).

Before lunch: Carrot juice.

Lunch Salad: Lettuce grated carrot, slices or two onions grated raw beetroot cress and mustard seeds.

Dressing dressing: chopped parsley and yogurt. 2 crisp rye breads and butter. Pear or apple to follow.

Mid-afternoon Herbal tea.

In the evening, before dinner After dinner, drink a glass of pineapple juice.

Evening dinner: Millet and Tomato Savoury with leeks and carrots. Apricots soaked in yogurt and soaked.

Wednesday

Breakfast Fruits for breakfast: fresh: grapes or pear.

Mid-morning: Vecon..

Before lunch: Pineapple juice.

LunchSalad lettuce tomatoes (skinned) grated carrot, 1/2 apple as well as sunflower seeds, watercress as well as raisins. Hard-boiled eggs. Oil dressing and cider vinegar.

Cut wholemeal bread into slices and spread butter. Apricots that have been baked.

Mid-afternoon Herbal tea.

In the evening, before dinner, drink Carrot juice.

Evening meal: Vegetables and Lentil Casserole with cabbage. Apple Crumble.

Thursday

Breakfast: Baked prunes, and Muesli.

The mid-morning hour: Barley Cup.

Before lunch: Apple juice.

Lunch: Brown Rice Salad.

Mid-afternoon Herbal tea.

Prior to dinner Before dinner: Carrot juice.

Evening dinner: Omelette (tomato or mushroom) along with peas (not canned) as well as carrots. Baked apple with raisins as well as fruitcake.

Friday

Breakfast: Two slices of of whole wheat toast and butter with honey.

Mid-morning: Vecon.

Before lunch: Apple juice.

Lunch: Brown Rice Salad.

Mid-afternoon Herbal tea.

In the evening, before dinner After dinner, drink a glass of carrot juice.

Evening dinner: Omelette (tomato or mushroom) and peas (not canned) as well as carrots and peppers stuffed with. Apples baked with raisins.

Saturday

Breakfast: Apricots boiled and yogurt.

The mid-morning hour: Barley Cup.

Lunch salad: lettuce tomatoes (skinned) cucumber (unskinned) chopped carrot, watercress 1/2 orange segmented and sunflower seeds. Vinaigrette dressing. Jacket potato baked and a bit of butter. Fresh fruit.

The mid-afternoon hours: China tea: Lapsang or jasmine.

Prior to dinner Before dinner: Carrot juice.

Evening meal: Chestnut Pudding with runners beans (in season) or greens of a kind and parsnips. Fruit Jelly.

Sunday

Breakfast: Toast, honey and butter.

Mid-morning: Tomato juice and the word "con.

Before lunch: Apple juice.

Lunch lunch: Cheesecake Soya Mix (page 90) broad beans, greens Mash turnips. Baked jacket potato. Fresh fruit salad, made from honey and yogurt.

In the afternoon, mid-afternoon. China or tea made from herbs.

Prior to dinner: Carrot juice.

Evening meal: Apple, pear, grapes; raisins (or dates), 12 almonds.

Monday

Breakfast: raw apple grated and muesli.

In the middle of the morning: tomato juice containing Vecon.

Before lunch: Apple juice.

Lunch: Coleslaw made of carrots and apple grated; cut cabbage and chopped onions (to the taste), raisins and sunflower seeds, served with a dressing made of yogurt as well as black pepper and cider vinegar (chopped mint could be added during the season). 2 breads with crisp rye and butter. Apricot crumble.

Mid-afternoon: Tea or China.

Prior to dinner After dinner, drink a glass of pineapple juice.

Dinner Start with a starter: Avocado with mint shaved along with lemon juice.

Second course The second course is Breakfast: Eggs and cheese Bake and carrots, runners beans, or cabbage.

Dessert Fresh or baked apple, or fruit.

Tuesday

Breakfast: Prunes or Apricot and yogurt. Rye crisp bread with butter, honey and butter.

In the middle of the morning: Barley Cup.

Before lunch: Carrot juice.

Lunch Salad: Lettuce, the watercress leaves, celery chopped, the pepper (green or red) and grated carrot, apple

Parsley chopped almonds, ground parsley (2 teaspoons). Baked

jacket potato, Vinaigrette dressing.

The Bread and Butter Pudding.

Mid-afternoon Tea: As usual. '

Before evening meal: Tomato juice.

Evening meal: Aduki Bean Hotpot, green vegetable.

Pineapple (fresh or canned in the natural juice).

Wednesday

Breakfast: Fruit: apple, orange, dates, almonds.

Mid-morning: tomato juice with Vecon as well as Barmene.

Before lunch: Pineapple juice.

Lunch Salad: Cottage cheese made with diced celery, grated carrots, cut parsley, raisins all served with watercress sprigs. Bread and butter made from wholemeal. Stewed apple.

Mid-afternoon: Tea.

In the evening, before dinner, drink Carrot juice.

Evening meal: First course: Avocado Vinaigrette.

Second course Second course and Cheese Bake served with jacket potatoes and the green vegetable (runner beans during the season).

Dessert The dessert can be fruit jelly or a fruit cake.

Thursday

Breakfast Raisins and Branflakes. 1 apple.

The mid-morning hour: Barley Cup.

Before lunch: Pineapple juice.

LunchSalad lettuce and watercress, tomato grated carrot, cucumber and sunflower seeds. Yogurt Mint Dressing. Grated Cheshire cheese (55 grams). Fresh fruit.

Mid-afternoon: tea or fruit juice.

Prior to dinner A good option is to drink carrot or tomato juice.

Evening meal: Lentil Roast (page 93), leeks, green vegetables. Baked apples and raisins.

Friday

Breakfast: V2 grapefruit, 1 pear, 8 dates, 8 almonds.

Yogurt.

Mid-morning: con, and tomato juice.

Before lunch: Pineapple juice.

Lunch: Watercress arid fresh orange segments served with almonds and yogurt. Bread with a crisp rye. Butter and bread pudding.

Mid-afternoon: Tea , or juice from fruit.

Prior to dinner After dinner, drink a glass of carrot juice.

Evening meal: Stuffed peppers. Parsnips or carrots, green vegetables. Apricots or prunes that are soaked.

Saturday

Breakfast: two slices of wholemeal toast Honey, butter, and butter. 1 apple.

The mid-morning hour: Barley Cup.

Before lunch: Pineapple juice.

Dinner: rice salad and watercress. Breads made of rye. Stewed apple.

Mid-afternoon Then tea (China or herbal).

Prior to dinner Before dinner: Carrot juice.

Evening meal: Savoury Jacket Potato, green vegetables. Juicy fruit and yogurt.

Sunday

Breakfast: Bran flakes and raisins. 1 apple.

The mid-morning hour: Barley Cup or Vecon.

Before lunch: Apple juice.

Lunch: Chestnut Pudding , carrots, green vegetables. Baked egg custard.

Mid-afternoon: The traditional coffee or cake with fruit.

Prior to dinner Before dinner: Carrot juice.

Evening dinner: Watercress. sandwiches. Dates, apples, pear and nuts.

These menus should have provided you with the knowledge to keep your diet on track. In addition to a potential increment in the amount however, the overall structure must remain the same. It is important not to boost the quantity excessively due to the possibility that an overly full stomach can protrude out of the Oesophageal opening. By avoiding pressure and eating nutritious, healthy foods, the likelihood of healing the hernia is greatly enhanced.

Chapter 4: Exercise

It was mentioned in an earlier article that exercising does more than keep muscles in good shape and in good shape, but also affects the tissues of the body through regular cell activity. The short bursts of exercise not beneficial; and simply doing just a few exercises for ten minutes a day is enough to keep your body flexible (though it's good) but without any more profound impact in cell function. This is the deeper effect that is essential to treat hiatus hernia and also for enhancing the abdominal muscle's endurance.

A walk in the park is ideal to accomplish this. It should last for at 30 to 40 minutes at a minimum before extending to an hour as much as is it is possible. In the beginning there may be a need for some people to be extra careful. It's a mistake to embark on a lengthy walk if not fully prepared for it. A normal walk, for instance for 20 minutes, has worth, and it could be gradually extended. It is better than going for a longer exercise only to be exhausted and being discouraged from undertaking any further. When done in this manner the walking process produces a subtle glowing or sweat that suggests that the entire system is working, and the elimination process is speeded up through the skin and lungs and leaves less harmful substances that clog the body.

Eliminating waste is essential to maintaining health. It is because many people aren't aware of this fact in all its aspects or are taught to observe bowel movements and ignore the skin and lungs that over-loading is a common occurrence. The bowel's action is often inadequate also, unfortunately. If a healthy eating plan and regular exercise is followed, the inequalities can be rebalanced by the inherent cell-types of our body which are health-focused.

The body is always striving to be healthy. If we could only be taught not to put spanners in the process due to poor diet and bad habits in general the amount of good health would be more high.

There are a variety of specific exercises designed for abdominal muscles. These are beneficial if done regularly and in a regular manner. It is probably advisable to gradually increase the duration in those unable or inexperienced to exercise. However, generally speaking, 15 to 20 minutes a day is the recommended duration needed to achieve maximum results. (The most crucial exercise - deep diaphragmatic breathing has been described.)

It is recommended to practice these exercises for ten minutes initially, before with, then increasing it to 20 minutes in time, will not only help you however, it will also improve awareness of your body and improve posture. We often do this because of fatigue, speed and the effects from gravity we can be prone to fall and slump while remaining tight while doing it. It is crucial to be aware of this and get up. Exercise can have both a physical as well as a mental impact, and can be of huge value.

But, don't move to the other side and become stiff in the stretched-up position! Do not lift your ribs gently by lowering and relaxing your shoulders, stretching the neck's back and the top of the head effortlessly. It instantly gives you a sense of increased control and integration , and the capacity to deal with the everyday round. If you feel like you are to earth' get your body up and remember the slow breathing. The same kind of exercise works in case you feel anxious and "up tight".

It's surprising how much is possible to do in order to avoid diseases and improve health. Health awareness is an exciting challenge and an opportunity to continue education and personal development.

Exercise 1:

Place yourself in a crook posture which is to say, with the knees bent, feet near buttocks, and arms spread to the sides. Put your hands on the thighs so that they meet the abdomen, then lift them until they reach the knees. raising the shoulders and head and inhaling slowly. Breathe out ,then fall back and taking a moment of relaxation. Repeat the exercise four up to 6 times. Watch the abdominal muscles contract as you push toward the ceiling.

Exercise 2:

Relax on your back and lie flat on your stomach with your legs straight. Bring both legs up to 45deg, breathe in slowly, and then lower them slowly, breathing out and relax. Repeat four times.

Exercise 3:

Sit on a stooland place your hands resting on the hips. Make use of your arms as levers turning initially to the right, then left. This motion is done at waist level. Take a look at each shoulder while you turn. In a way, if you count a left and right turn as one the sequence seven to 10 times. Do not do any breathing exercises, but be aware that you don't need to hold your breath.

Exercise 4:

Sit in a straight-backed chair with your back supported and your the bottom well-tucked back with arms resting on the side. Breathe out and relax forward. (head down to the knees). Uncurl and push your back against to the rear of your chair, until you are upright and breathing slowly all the time. Be sure to keep your head lower until the position of upright is reached. The back should be round and not curling. Don't come upwards in a straight line. Repeat four times.

Exercise 5:

This exercise is designed to raise the rib cage and widen the chest. As in Exercise 4, sit down. Place hands behind your neck and lean forward, and bend your elbows toward knees. Then raise your back, bracing elbows (parallel to shoulder muscles) and breathing into. Releasing forward breathe out and let the elbows slide forward. Re-inflate as you did you can before. You will feel the ribs lifting! Repeat the exercise four to six times.

Exercise 6:

This is designed to improve the chest and spine to move. In a 'donkey' posture - on all fours with arms and thighs at right angles to your body with the with the spine straight. Then, bend your head downwards. At the same time, hump your spine (so that everything is round) and breathe into. Change your posture by 'hollowing' your lower back, and then raising the head to the side. Breathe in as you do this. Keep your elbows straight as the thighs and arms serve as the pillars of support. Six times repeat.

Chapter 5: Additional Natural

Treatments

Hydrotherapy

Water is a potent source of natural healing, which is often overlooked. Cold water may be a tonic for nerves and blood vessels especially on the skin. Warm water can relax the body, but must be handled with care. The cold and hot water utilized in contrast, is extremely stimulating and helpful in speeding removal, absorption and healing. Ice is beneficial for treating injuries that have occurred recently, and also prevents the body from over-reacting to injury. The cold compresses on the area offer a natural warm sensation, that relaxes the body and aids in removal and absorption of harmful matter. Self-generated warmth is superior over heat applied to the body from outside. Water is extremely beneficial in controlling body temperature through applying complete body packs to encourage sweating or splashing to lower temperatures that are high.

Water was used for therapeutic purposes since ancient times. The Greeks and Romans recognized its benefits externally as well as internally. They invented a method of colonic lavage using the horn of an animal to transport the water to the rectum. Thus, colonic washouts and enemas are not new!

Additionally, there are or were spa towns, which were places in which people would go to 'take the waters' - either for drinking it soak in it or both. Unfortunately, many of the English spas have been shut down however those on the continent appear to be kept.

The application of water in the event of hiatus hernia is in shape of cold compresses applied to the abdomen's upper region. The reason for these is because the packs promote an increase in circulation temporarily in the region of the stomach and diaphragm and, consequently, enhances their performance. Furthermore, the absorption process of cell waste matter is increased and muscle tone is enhanced.

The pack is put on for at least three hours, but should be put on before bed and worn throughout the night. The first effect of the cold substance on the skin and subcutaneous tissues results in an increase in the size of blood vessels. It is then followed by dilation. This is supported by more extensive vessels and overall activity in the area is activated. Following the initial jolt on the cold that is expected to be only a few seconds the skin should feel very at ease and pleasantly warm. The frequency of treatment is at least two times each week, or every day, for three weeks, prior to the beginning of treatment.

To make an Ice Pack:

You'll need between four and six layers of linen or cotton (old sheets or towelling) 18cm square.

A piece of woollen material , or flannelette. It measures 23 cm square.
A large towel folded lengthways, to function as binder.
Three large safety pins.
Method:
Soak the cotton in cold water. Then wring it out until it is damp. and smooth out any wrinkles. Apply to the abdomen's upper part and smooth out any creases. This is the area where the ribs separate between them, and also the umbilicus (navel). Cover the area with the bigger piece of material and ensure that there is a good contacts with skin and then bind by folding the towel firm but not too tight. Put the pin in place: put on your nightwear and then go to the bed.
The pack should feel warm (or not even cold) If it does it does not, two errors could be made. (1) Pack might not have been drained enough; (2) contact may be weak and air could be getting into the skin and the pack. If none of these are the situation it means that the body's

energy isn't strong enough to respond properly, and the pack needs to be discarded and tested at a later time in the treatment, perhaps within two weeks. It is crucial that the pack warms up and doesn't remain cold and clammy. It can only be effective if it gets warm within the first 10 minutes after application. If this is not the case then it must be removed.

Note: No waterproofing product is recommended, since it alters the function of the pack and turns to a lotion which is not the result intended. When the pack is taken off within the timeframe of three hours or morning, as the case is, the skin as well as the material of the pack should be rinsed with warm water to get rid of any trace of harmful matter. This should be eliminated by the skin and pack.

There are a variety of ways that water can be used to help with healing and one of them is to complete the hot shower or bath by soaking in a cold shower. Start with your feet and legs, they are the least sensitive parts then move on to the abdomen, arms and back. This can be accomplished with sponges, a few drops of water, or with a shower attachment. Then, finish with a quick massage using a rough towel. Your entire body will appear glowing and alive.

Additional Information for Use During Temporary Periods

Vitamin E Wheatgerm oil capsules assist in healing as well as the efficient utilization of oxygen in bloodstream (100 IU of strength but not more than 3 capsules daily). Discontinue after six weeks.

Herbal tranquilizers: To aid in relief from anxiety, insomnia or general anxiety, consider a herb tranquilizer, which contains some Vitamin B Complex that helps the nervous system is a possibility.

Tissue Salts Biochemical trace elements that help activate and balance bodily functions are essential in treating hiatus hernia. Calcium fluoride which increases elasticity, is especially beneficial in this instance. These salts are available in pharmacies for health foods and are taken according to the directions. Both the tissue salts as well as the herbal tranquilizers are recommended for use for more than two months. However, should it be necessary, one or both may be reintroduced following a period of time. The main goal on natural remedies is to reduce the necessity of taking medications and adjust your entire lifestyle to maintain a healthy balance and equilibrium.

Chapter 6: Recipes

Breakfasts

HOME-MADE MUSELI

455 g of oat wheat or barley flake

115 g raw cane sugar

115 g raisins

115 g chopped hazel nuts

55 g of dried milk powder

8 dried apricots that have been dried, chopped smaller

1 raw apple with a grated

1 Combine dry ingredients ready to use. Store in an airtight tin container.

2 Serve with a grated apple. It is recommended to soak each piece in water overnight and then add the apple the next morning.

FRUIT and NUT FRUIT AND NUT

1 sweet apple

1 dessertspoon raisins

1 teaspoon sunflower seeds

1 dessertspoon of ground almonds

1 Thoroughly wash the apple then grate the apple with a coarse grated (skin and

core also) and then place in bowl. Add other ingredients, mixing somewhat.

2. Eat slowly and chew your food thoroughly!

FRUITY YOGURT

115 g raisins , sultanas or sultan

1 large grapefruit or orange

140 ml natural yogurt

1 Wash the raisins and remove them from bowl. Pour boiling water until it is covered with a stir. Allow to soak for a night.

2. In the morning, peel the orange and then remove the pith. Cut thinly using a an abrasive knife.

3 Place in a dish and add raisins that are soaked in yogurt and the.

Main Meals

CHESTNUT and COURGETTE SAVOURY

Serves 2

3-4 medium courgettes

2 Tablespoons of sunflower oil

Whole chestnuts tinned to 115g

Pinch salt from the sea

1 teaspoon of dried herbs mixed with

2 eggs, beaten

Fresh parsley chopped to 1 tablespoon

1 Clean and dry the courgettes. Slice thinly.

2 2: Heat the sunflower oil inside a fry pan. Add the courgettes cut into pieces and toss around to brown them. add the chestnuts you've rinsed and stir to warm them up and then add dried herbs and salt.

3 Pour the batter over the eggs, then lower the heat and allow it to set. Sprinkle with chopped parsley.

4 . Serve it with baked jacket potatoes and carrots.

NUTTY BEAN BAKE

Serves 3

Whole chestnuts 115 grams

55 g hazelnuts that have been coarsely ground

55 g sunflower or pumpkin seeds

55 g of wholemeal breadcrumbs

1/2 teaspoon of thyme

Aduki beans 115 grams, that were soaked for a night

1 medium carrot grated

2 eggs

Pinch salt from the sea

1 Mix the seeds, nuts breadcrumbs, herbs ingredients. Drain the Aduki beans and add as well as the grated carrot.

2. Add the eggs, one at a and mix well with the seasoning. Pour into a baking dish.

3 Bake in a medium-sized oven at 375 degF/190degC for 35 to 45 minutes. Enjoy with salad as well as Carrot Sauce (opposite).

CARROT SAUCE

1 Mix 2 medium-sized carrots using juice from one lemon and 1 pinch sea salt.

2 Place in pan and cook Add 1 teaspoon of agar powder (Gelozone) and bring to boiling while stirring.

3 Pour the sweet sauce over and serve.

SAVOURY Apple PUDDING

Serves 3-4

115 g sunflower margarine

55 g ground almonds

115 g of wholemeal breadcrumbs

115 g of wholemeal plain flour

2 eggs, beaten

Freshly ground black pepper and Sea Salt

1 teaspoon of dried sage

1 Bramley apple with coarsely grated

1 small onion Finely chopped

1. Soften and cream margarine. Add the almonds ground up along with the crumbled crumbs, and flour.

2. Add eggs, salt onion, sage and apple Mix well.

3 Place in a basin that is greased, then be covered with greaseproof paper and a tying down cloth and then steam for

1 1/2 hours.

4 . Serve warm with broccoli, apples and carrots. It can be served cold, with salad.

MILLET and TOMATO SAVOURY

Serves 1

2 oz (55 g) millet

A small-sized tin (7 200 g/200 oz) tomatoes

1 clove of garlic crushed

2 tablespoons mix herbs

1/2 teaspoon yeast extract

1 Mix all ingredients in a pan made of steel and cook gently until the millet is able to absorb all of the water.

2. Stir regularly.

3 Serve with fresh vegetables.

BAKE CHEESE AND EGG

Serves 2

2 eggs

425 ml milk

1 tablespoon mixed herb

55 grams grated Cheddar cheese

1) Beat the eggs thoroughly. Add milk and mix in all the ingredients.

2 Pour the batter into an oven-proof dish. Set it in a bigger pan that has 1 centimeter of water.

3 Bake at 350degF/180degC in 45 mins or till it is set.

CHEESY SOYA MIX

Serves 2

One small onion cut into slices

1 cup sunflower seed oil

1 carrot grated

55 g soya flakes

30 g ground almonds

55 G Cheddar cheese grated

1 egg, beaten

1 teaspoon mixed herbs or sage

Mixing the water If necessary, mix the water.

1 . Lightly cook the onions in oil. Take it off the stove.

2. Mix all dry ingredients in the bowl.

3 Mix in the onion, and then add the egg that has been beat.

4. If the mix isn't enough to be able to stick together, you can add a few drops of water.

5 Cook using one of the methods below:

* Make into rissoles, then fry with only a tiny amounts of oil.

* Pour the batter into an ovenproof dish lightly oiled and bake at 375 degF/190 degC (Gas Mark 5) for 25 to 35 minutes.

Pour the mixture into an oily bowl. It is then covered using greaseproof newspaper and let it steam for 30 to 40 minutes.

VEGETABLE and LENTIL CASSEROLE
Serves 2

1 onion, or leek chopped

1 tablespoon of oil (sunflower, soya , or olive)

2 big carrots chopped into small

2 sticks of celery cut into pieces

2 small turnips or 1 tiny Swede, chopped small

4 cabbage leaves to be chopped

1 vegetable stock cube

1 teaspoon Vecon

285 milliliters boiling water

4 bay leaves

1 tablespoon mixed herb

Four tablespoons of Lentils (green or dark)

1. Cook the onions (or Leeks) in oil until it is lightly brown. In a casserole, include the rest of the vegetables.

2 Heat the cubes of stock as well as Vecon into the water. Add bay leaves and herbs, then sprinkle over the vegetables.

3 Drain the lentils through a sieve that is drained under the tap. Add to the casserole. Mix well. The ingredients

should be covered with liquid in case not, add a bit additional hot water.

4 Cover and bake on the stove at 350 degF/180 degC for 1 1/2 hours.

ADUKI BEAN HOTPOT

Serves 2

1 onion

110 grams Aduki beans

3-4 carrots

1 Tablespoon tomato paste

1 vegetable stock cube

560 ml boiling water

1 tablespoon oil

1/4 teaspoon sea salt (optional)

1 Slice the onion , and fry in oil until it is browned. Sesame seeds for garnish Place in a casserole dish.

2 Rinse aduki beans and place in a saucepan that is covered with water and bring to a boil. Cook for 5 minutes after which you can drain and dispose of the water.

3. Place the beans in the pot along with the onion.

Four Chop your carrots in small pieces and add them the carrots to the pot.

5 Dissolve the cubes of stock in boiling water, then add the tomato puree, then add the other ingredients.

Make sure the seasoning is in order. If the cube of stock was unseasoned, you might have to add some salt.

6. Bake in a 325oF/140oC oven, for 1 1/2 hours.

Variation:

Mung beans can be substituted for Aduki beans.

LENTIL ROAST

120 g green or brown lentils cooked

30 g ground almonds

1 slice of wholemeal bread with a crumbled

1 onion, cut into slices

3 tablespoons of oil

1 carrot

2 tablespoons mix herbs

1 teaspoon of sea salt

Black pepper freshly ground

1 egg, beaten

Sesame seeds as garnish

1 Mix the almonds, breadcrumbs, and lentils together.

2 Fry the onion slices in 1 tablespoon of oil until it is browned. add it to the mixture.

3 Coarsely grated your carrots into the mix Add the herbs, as well as the remaining oil. Mix thoroughly.

4 Add seasoning , and beat egg, and mix again.

5 Pour into a loaf tin lightly oiled. Press it down and trace the top with the help of a fork. Bake at

350degF/190degC for 35 mins followed by a time at 400degF/200degC 20 minutes.

6 Transfer to an uncooked plate, and sprinkle using sesame seeds.

CHESTNUT PUDDING

4 oz/115 g chestnut puree

45 G wholemeal breadcrumbs

1 small tin (7200 g) tomatoes

Two teaspoons of mixed herb

A pinch of sea salt, as well as freshly crushed black pepper

2 tablespoons soya-based flour

1 small egg; beaten

1. Mix all ingredients in a bowl (if too dry, make sure you add a bit extra soya powder) Then, pour the mix in a basin that has been greased.

2 Cover this with an apron then steam for an hour.

3 Pour the pudding onto a serving dish and serve. The dessert looks nice set in an oblong ring of mashed carrots and is great to eat warm with vegetables or cold with salad.

Snacks along with Light Meals

SAVOURY JACKET POTATO

(Ingredients for each person)

1/2 onion

1 tomato, skinned

130 grams of grated Cheshire cheese

A small amount of vegetable oil

1 hot baked potato

1 Slice onion into slices and fry until it becomes translucent. Slice tomatoes in

half and cook for 2 mins while frying the onion.

2 Add the cheese at the very last minute to melt slightly.

3 Cut the potato in half, pour in the filling. Double it again, and serve it with green vegetables.

TOMATOES and ONIONS on TOAST

1 Peel and scale 2 tomatoes, then slice them. chop and peel one small onion.

2 Place a knob of margarine in a skillet and let it melt. Then add the onion chopped, and roast lightly.

3 Add diced tomatoes and a teaspoon of mixed herbs. Cook for 3-5 minutes.

4 Prepare 1 or two slices of toasted wholemeal bread. Layer the onion and tomato mixture on top of it and eat!

STUFFED PEPPERS

(Ingredients in a person)

One medium-sized, pepper (red or green)

1 tablespoon brown rice 1 tablespoon brown

1 clove garlic that has been crushed

2 teaspoons mixed herbs

1 carrot grated

4 dried apricots, cut into pieces

1 Cut off the tops of peppers, and then remove the seeds and the core. Have an oven tin prepared with 2 cm of water to place the peppers in.

2 Wash and cook it in salted and steamed water for around 15 minutes. Then remove and mix it with the garlic, herb, carrots and apricots.

3. Stuff the mixture into the bell peppers, and cook for about 40-50 mins at 375degP/190degC , in central oven. Sprinkle the seasoning lightly.

AVOCADO and CREAM CHEESE WHICH IS ADDED WITH MINT

Serves 2

1 Halve an avocadoand Sprinkle with vinegar and stuff it with 55g of cream cheese.

2. Sprinkle the mint with chopped (generously) and a second shake with cider vinegar.

3 Eat Wholemeal Bread and Butter.

Simple TOMATO SAUCE AND SPAGHETTI

Serves 2

115 g of wholewheat spaghetti

200 g tomato tin

1 clove of garlic

1 teaspoon Barbados sugar

Pinch salt from the sea

1 teaspoon of agar

1. Boil spaghetti in the usual manner in salted water according to the instructions on the packet.

2 Make Tomato Sauce: Empty tin into a small pan and chop tomatoes. Add sugar and garlic. Heat to a boil, then add the agar. Cook for 1 minute.

3. Serve with the spaghetti.

Salads

CHICORY, ORANGE and AVOCADO "SUNRISE"

1 Cut an avocado in half and remove the flesh from the skin. Slice into cubes.

2. Peel the orange. then slice it thickly then cut it into pieces. mix in avocado and then pile on top of a small dish.

3 Lay out chicory leaves (like sun Rays) to be incorporated into the mix.

Four Sprinkle some chopped mint on top the salad if you're feeling fancy. Serve with butter and wholemeal bread.

PINEAPPLE and APPLE, AND GINGER SALAD

3 apples

3 pieces of stem ginger

Tin pineapple weighing 340 grams with its juice

1 lettuce 1 lettuce, washed

1 bunch watercresswashed, rinsed

Vinaigrette (recipe coming up)

1 teaspoon yogurt mixed in 1 tablespoon of sugar.

pineapple juice (more if necessary)

1 teaspoon chopped mint

Flaked almonds

1 Finely chop apples Chop ginger. Cut pineapple (if in rings) into chunks.

2 Tear the lettuce, sprinkle with sprigs watercress and mix with French dressing. Distribute on a platter.

3 Mix apple, pineapple and ginger into the yogurt as well as the juice of pineapple. Place on the base of watercress and lettuce Sprinkle with almonds and mint.

BRUSSELS SPROUTS and CELERY, AND Apple SALAD

1 Serve 4 large sprouts two sticks of celery, and 1 apple per person.

2. Make Dessert Salad Dressing.

3 On a cutting board using an incredibly sharp knife cut celery and sprouts coarsely or finely as you like.

4 Grate the apple finely Mix the salad ingredients, then add dressing and decorate with sunflower seeds or sultanas.

BETROOT AND CELERY SALAD

1 Prepare Cottage Cheese Dressing.

2 Peel 2 beetroots that have been cooked (globe kind are the best tasting) cut and dice them and place into a large dish.

3 Pick a head of celery, cut relatively small, omitting the hard outer sticks.

4 - Mix beetroot with Add more celery if you prefer beetroot.

5 Add the dressing from Cottage Cheese The mixture will change to pink.

6 Serve a spoonful of salad on the watercress or lettuce.

SPROUTED SALAD

Alfalfa or bean sprouts

Young dandelion leaves

Young nasturtium leaves

Mint or chives to enhance the flavour

Vinaigrette

1 Mix all ingredients of the salad in vinaigrette. To add a pop of colour grated carrots or sliced tomatoes can be added.

Salad Dressings

COTTAGE DRESSING WITH CHEESE

115 g cottage cheese

1 clove of garlic crushed

2-3 fresh sage leaves, chopped finely

Three tablespoons of cider vinegar

1 teaspoon sunflower oil

1 Mix everything in one container and then refrigerate until you need it.

BROWN RICE SALAD

(Serves 2)

115 grams brown rice washed

1 Tablespoon vegetable oil

1 glove garlic crushed

1 large carrot grated

1/2 green pepper Finely chopped

1 teaspoon fresh chopped mint (or chives)

1 apple, diced

A handful of raisins

2 sticks of celery, chopped

1/2 bunch watercress, washed and finely chopped

2 tablespoons finely cut or ground nuts your choice

1/2 bunch of watercress, washed to garnish

1 Bring 850ml salted water to the point of boiling and then add the rice along with the oil and minced garlic.

2 Cook for 35 minutes with stirring from time to the time. Drain in a sieve or colander before allowing to cool.

3 Once the rice is cool - add the other ingredients and mix thoroughly. Serve with the rest of the watercress for garnish.

VINAIGRETTE

2 Tablespoons of cider vinegar

1 teaspoon sunflower seeds oil

1 . cloves of garlic crushed

1/2 to 1 teaspoon of honey

Any herb, for flavor

1. Mix the ingredients.

2 Eat with any kind of salad, or avocado 3 Serve with pears.

SWEET SALAD DRESSING

3 Tablespoons vinegar from cider

1 Tablespoon sunflower oil

1 teaspoon honey

1 tablespoon mild mustard

1 tablespoon juice of pineapple

1 Mix all the liquids together or put it into an screw-top bottle or jar with a vigorous shake.

YOGURT MINT DRESSING

1 teaspoon mint

140 ml natural yogurt

1 teaspoon honey

1. Mix the ingredients.

2 Serve alongside salads.

Desserts

1. APPLE CRUMBLE 1.

(Serves 2)

2 cooking apples

1 dessertspoon raw sugar from cane

1 lemon. Grated the rind, and juice

100 percent 115g wholemeal flour

1 table-spoon raw sugar from cane

55 g of unsalted butter

1 . Core and slice the apple and then grate them, with the skin, into a ovenproof dish.

2 Mix the juice, grated zest of the lemon, as well as the sugar. Mix well.

3 Cover this mix with sugar, flour, and margarine, which are mixed and then rubbed to create fine breadcrumbs.

4 Press lightly over the mixture of apples.

5 Bake the cake at 200degF/400degF in 20-30 minutes.

APPLE CRUMBLE 2

(Serves 2)

Apple Mix

Three large cooking apples

Squeeze cloves, cinnamon, or lemon rinds grated to enhance the flavor

2 tablespoons raw raw dark sugar

1. Peel and cut the apples. Arrange in a baking dish.

2. Sprinkle the flavoring of your choice, according to preference, along with the sugar.

Topping

3 heaped tablespoons of 100 percent wholemeal flour

1 tablespoon raw cane sugar

I use a tablespoon of ground almonds.

85 g of unsalted butter

1 Mix the dry ingredients and cut them into the butter. Rub it in until you have an even breadcrumb texture.

2. Sprinkle the apples to create the crust. Press it down gently. Bake at 400degF/200degC for 30-40 mins.

SULTANA SCONES

115 g sunflower margarine

Wholemeal Plain Flour 225g

55 g soft raw cane sugar

55 g sultanas

Mix yogurt and milk

2 Rub butter into flour, until it resembles breadcrumbs, then cut into Sultanas, sugar.

2. Mix 1 tablespoon of milk and 1 dessert spoon natural yogurt to moisten the dry mix by stirring it using the help of a knife. If needed, add more liquid until you reach the point where the dough is able to be kneaded into a smooth ball.

3 Spread on the board with flour. Using fingers, press it out until 1.5-2 millimeters in thickness.

Be aware that since there is no raising agent the scones will be exactly the same size as they were when baked.

4 Cut it out using a pastry cutter , then bake in the oven to 400 degrees F/200 degrees C for 25 minutes.

FLAPJACKS

170 g sunflower margarine

Black treacle 115 grams

55 g Demerara sugar

250 g of Oats rolled

55 g of hazelnuts, walnuts or hazelnuts

115 g sultanas

1 Melt butter, sugar and treacle gently in a pan. Then, mix in the rest of the ingredients. Mix well.

2 Transfer onto a baking tin that is greased Press down evenly then bake the cake at 375degC or 190degC for 30 to 35 minutes.

3 Cut into fingers or squares while still hot. Cool on a wire tray. When it is cold cut into pieces.

STEAMED SULTANA PUDDING

(Serves 2)

55 g of unsalted butter

55 g dark raw cane sugar

1 large egg, beaten

100 percent 115g wholemeal plain flour

The rind of one lemon is grated.

55 g of sultanas well cleaned

1 Lightly oil a pudding dish.

2 Mix the sugar and butter and beat into the egg, then add the flour, lemon rind. Add the sultanas. Mix should have a

drop-like consistency. If it's the mixture is too stiff, mix in a bit of water and lemon juice.

3 Pour into the basin and cover with greaseproof paper and cloth and tie securely or use a lid if the basin comes with one. Place in pan with 5cm boiling water, about halfway up sides of the basin. It should simmer for about an hour. Top it off with boiling water more intervals and keep it at the halfway point.

4 . Serve it with a sprinkle of sunflower seeds or sesame seeds.

BREAD and BUTTER PUDDING
(Serves 2)
2 large slices of wholemeal bread with butter
55 g raisins or sultanas Well cleaned
1 egg, beaten
285 ml milk
1 tablespoon raw sugar from cane

1 Lightly butter the oven-safe dish. Slice butter and bread to cover the sides and the bottom of the dish.

Sprinkle it with raisins or sultanas.

2 Mix the egg, sugar and milk together, then pour it over.

3 3 Bake in the oven at 350degF/180degC (Gas Mark 4) for 40 minutes. Then, increase the temperatures to 400oF/200oC and bake for 10 minutes, in order to cook the top of the pudding.

FRUIT JELLY

It can be made using fresh or dried fruit. Apples and bananas, oranges, pears either in combination or singly with raisins, prunes, apricots that have been previously soaked.

1. Prepare the fruit in small dishes or bowls - either chop or coarsely grate the pear or apple. cut the banana in thick slices or pear; cut it into segments and then the orange. .

2 For every 285 ml liquid (water or juice) you'll require an equal amount of agar-agar, or Gelozone. The liquid needs to be heated and then allowed to rest for a

few minutes before pouring it over the fruit.

3 The powder used to make the jelly may be made into a paste with cold water, and the remaining added slowly or sprinkled over the warm water as it warms up - not until it is boiling.

4 Honey or sugar may be added according to the taste.

Be aware that these jellies won't serve on a plate very well , so small plates or large bowls is ideal.

ALMOND CAKE

115 g sunflower margarine (or similar)

2 Tablespoons of sunflower oil

115 g soft raw cane sugar

3 eggs

170 g of wholemeal plain flour

55 g soya flour

55 g ground almonds

2-5 drops of almond essence natural (optional)

55g flaked almonds

1. Prepare an 18cm cake in a tin.

2. In a large bowl or mixer, blend the oil, fat and sugar.

Three eggs should be added one after one, and add a bit from the flours (which have been sifted along with the almonds that have been ground) to avoid curdling.

4 Fold into the remaining flour mix. Add the essence (if you are using it) and half of the almonds that have been flaked.

5 Pour into the tin that you have prepared The middle should be hollow to allow for rising and sprinkle on the rest of the almonds that have been flaked.

6 Bake in the centre of oven at 375 degF/190degC for one 1/2 hours. Cover with greaseproof papers, but take it off for the final half hour.

Variation: This mix can be used to create tiny buns, by making use of Patty Tins.

Old-fashioned rich fruit cake

Unsalted butter 115 grams

55 g sunflower margarine

2 Tablespoons of sunflower oil

55 g soft raw cane sugar

1 tablespoon honey with light flavour.

Wholemeal Plain Flour 225g

55 g soya flour

55 g ground almonds

4 eggs

The juice and rinse of 1 large lemon

115 g sultanas

55 G currants

115 g raisins

55 grams chopped Apricots

Flaked almonds for decoration

1. Prepare an 18cm cake Tin.

2 Mix the butter, margarine sugar, oil and honey.

3 Sift the almonds and flour together, but don't add them to the creamed mix yet.

4 Beat eggs, slowly mix the eggs with the creamed mixture, adding some flour to stop curdling. Continue to add eggs until all are added.

5. Now fold in the rest of the flour, then grate in the lemon rind , and then add the juice. Add the fruit and mix well using the lifting (folding) motion. The consistency should be soft dropping, i.e.,

it falls off the spoon easily and is not too moist.

6 Transfer the mixture to a baking pan. Sprinkle almonds flakes on top.

7. Cover the baking pan with greaseproof papers and bake at a medium oven at 350 degF/180degC for an hour Remove the cover and increase temperature to 375degF/190degC over 30-40 minutes.

Notice: An alteration in flavor is possible with black treacle in place of honey. You can also substitute two teaspoons mixed spice in place of the lemon's rind (the juice will be required).

CAKE FOR LUNCH

1 Cup All Bran

1 Cup mixed fruits

1/2 cup soft brown sugar

1 cup milk

1 cup of wholemeal or rice flour

1 egg

1. Soak all Bran, mixed fruit and sugar overnight. All Bran, mixed fruit and sugar overnight in milk.

2 The next day, mix into the flour and beat egg.

3 Bake in a loaf pan at 350degF/180degC, for 45 minutes.

Note: Very delicious spread when paired with butter or margarine.

Miscellaneous:

Making Juices using a Juicer

This method can be used to prepare root vegetables, or any fruit that is able to be grate. You'll need the soup plate or dish, as well as a piece of gauze or muslin that's about 35cm in size, as well as grated.

1 Arrange the muslin inside the dish, and then grate the fruit or vegetable into it, then pull up the muslin with care and squeeze the pulp's juice.

2. Transfer the juice into an mug or cup and dilute it with a tablespoon of water. Drink (sip) in one go. (100 milliliters is the minimum amount.)

Note Be aware that beetroot, carrot and apples can be used, though maybe less often, due to their unique flavor, as are swede, potato and turnip.

Spouting Seeds Grains, Beans

1 Use a glass container that is covered with gauze, and secured with an elastic band.

2 Place about 1 dessert spoonful of any grains or seeds you want to use into the jar. Then wash thoroughly with cold water . No remains should be left inside the jar.

3 Place the gauze on the lid. Every day, clean the seeds (it is possible to do this through the lid and not remove it) and drain the water well.

4 Sprouts are visible within 3 to 6 days. They will increase to 2.5-4 cm. Remove them from the jar. You can eat both the seeds as well as the sprouts.

5. Repeat the process.

There are many examples to consider:

Beans

Aduki

Mung

Chickpeas

Soya

Haricot

Black-eyed

Seeds

Alfalfa

Mustard

Cress

Fennel

Sesame

Beet

Carrot

Grains

Wheat

Rye

Barley

Tips on food Combinations

Certain vegetables are known for causing problems in the digestive tract. And naturally, the cause varies between individuals However, the most common culprits are:

Cauliflower

Brussels Sprouts

Onions

Parsnips

Turnips

Cucumber

The first two vegetables should be cooked in a low temperature, to prevent the excessive production of sulphur in these vegetables that is the source of the problem within the body. If any of these vegetables are consumed, it is best to not serve potatoes at the same time.

All meat proteins and potatoes must be kept separate. If you are eating meat then carrots and vegetables are the most effective combination. Jacket potatoes can be enjoyed in salads, or with vegetarian dishes , but not pasta, since this is too concentrated in starch.

The mixture of fresh fruits and starch must be avoided as it causes gas and fermentation that destroys the vitamin content of the fruit and also slows absorption and digestion. Dry fruits and bananas however, are able to be mixed with starch.

The most frequently complained about are watercress, cucumbers and radishes.

When eaten in small amounts in a salad mix (using one of these at one time) and not drinking simultaneously the vegetables are digested easily provided they're chewed properly. There should not be problems if the suggestions regarding chewing is followed as well as certain recipes are used.

It is important to note that baking powder should not be utilized for any dish. I don't make use of baking powder or similar raising agents because they hinder the absorption of vitamin B and cause irritation to the digestive tract. Thus, recipes with baking powder are not recommended - or an egg can be substituted if it is suitable. This is an excellent reason to avoid cakes from shops and biscuits since they typically contain baking powder and other chemicals to enhance flavour and colour.

Chapter 7: Hernia Causes

An inguinal hernia develops when this weakening of the inguinal canal allows for an opening to form, normally due to an increased pressure within the abdomen. The causes of the pressure to increase include:

Other symptoms are:

Heavy lifting

Lifting using the back rather than the legs

- Forced, difficult or strenuous constipation movements

Constipation that is frequent and often painful.

Chronic coughing

- Constant coughing

- Frequent standing for lengthy periods

All of them cause tension and pressure on the abdomen. Over time, this pressure could force tissue into the abdominal wall which can cause an abdominal hernia.

The symptoms and signs of the Hernia

It is possible for you to suffer from a hernia without apparent signs. Your doctor will be the only one to find this. Most of the time, however an inguinal hernia may be associated with one or more of the signs listed below.

The most typical symptoms of a hernia are the appearance of a bulge on the right or left part, as well as both that is in line with the pubic bone. It is possible to gently press it back into a flat after the bulge is put back in the place it belongs.

- The groin region is painful when bowel movements are strained.

Pain in the region of the groin when you cough or sneezing.

The pain or pressure can be felt in the groin after lifting large objects

There can be swelling and pain around the testicles

The amount of discomfort and pain that is associated with the hernia could range between moderate and mild. It can also become more severe in period of time, as the hernia gets bigger.

Hernia Pain Relief

There are two kinds of relief products that are available for those suffering from hernias: traditional pain relievers and those to keep the herniated tissue to where it belongs.

The products that relieve pain comprise Ibuprofen as well as Tylenol. The usual cautions apply. Read the label carefully and follow the directions or consult your doctor for a recommendation.

The other kind of products for relief from hernias are hernia Trusses. They are described below under the heading "Hernia Treatment without Surgery."

Hernia Risks Untreated

The first step is to realize that a hernia won't be repaired by it self. If medical problems are left untreated, they will get better with time. Hernias are not one of those medical conditions that heal themselves.

A hernia will not only not heal itself , but it could get worse as time passes if it is not treated. The lining tear will become bigger. If you choose to repair it surgically, the procedure will need a more extensive repair. A larger repair can be more painful as well as more complex. This is the primary reason that I chose to not defer the surgery.

Inmates Hernia

The intestine's loop could become trapped within the an abdominal wall. This is referred to as an hernia that has been incarcerated. It can result in:

The obstruction of the colon

- Extreme pain

- Nausea

- Vomiting

- Completely inability to experience the bowel movements

It's like pushing the kink out of the garden hose. There is nothing that can override the kink. If it's the digestive tract, not an irrigation hose, it could result in severe constipation and discomfort.

Strangulated Hernia

If an infected hernia is sufficient to stop the flow of blood to a portion of your intestine, it's known as a strangulated hernia. The condition could lead to the death of the tissue in your bowel affected.

It is a life-threatening condition that requires immediate emergency surgery. My surgeon informed me that while I was waiting for my procedure If I noticed symptoms of this condition, to visit the hospital's Emergency Room (ER) promptly and then call his number immediately. It could be very serious.

How to Tell

There's an easy test that will make it easier to determine whether you're suffering from this issue or not.

Just press down on the hernia protruding. It should be possible feel the organs protruding back inside when you press them, and the protrusion should shrink in size.

If they're feeling stuck and aren't able to move easily it is recommended that you visit the ER immediately.

If your organs are able to slide back in without difficulty, you'll be secured for now.

Other signs of strangulated hernias include:

- Inability to pass gas and to pass gas

Tenderness and redness in the region of the hernia bulge

A painful sensation that increases dramatically rapidly and never goes completely

The symptoms can be associated with nausea and vomiting.

If you think that you be suffering from a strangulated hernia, you should visit the nearest emergency room as soon as possible.

The Hernia Treatment Without Surgery

The scientific literature that is reputable appears to agree that the best treatment to treat an inguinal hernia, is surgery. Hernias don't heal by themselves.

I did read a story of a "holistic" cure offered by one man who claims to have had his hernia removed without surgery. If it did work or not didn't bother me as per his own words, it took more than sixteen years to achieve. At this point, he needed to limit his activities to avoid pressure on the abdominal region. In his own words, every time he believed that the problem cured, it would come back.

For me , that was not acceptable. I'd be unable to pick up, carry as well as playing with my kids for sixteen years? Then it'd be too for me to be.

It's not a problem for anyone to be choosing this method however for me, it wasn't an alternative.

There are methods, however to lessen the discomfort from the hernia , and also to stop it from becoming in size during the time of waiting for surgery.

Hernia Trusses

Although it is not a substitute for surgery for repair the hernia truss could offer some relief from the discomfort from the hernia. This is particularly the case when coughing, lifting or sneezing, or other actions that can make the hernia uncomfortable.

A hernia-truss is an undergarment that is designed to press down on the protruding tissue of the hernia, and keep the hernia in the right position. It can be of aid while waiting for a permanent fix with surgical repair for hernias.

Surgery Options

The good news is that the inguinal the repair of hernias is among of the most popular general surgical procedures performed in the world. In fact hundreds of thousands of surgeries are carried out each year. This means that the majority of general surgeon is likely to have a lot of knowledge of this procedure.

If you're thinking about surgery for your inguinal hernia repair , there are two options to be thought of:

- Non Mesh vs. Mesh
- Open Surgery in contrast to. Laparoscopic surgery

There are positives and negatives for each , and each should be carefully considered.

Non Mesh Hernia Repair

This is an open surgical procedure. An incision of about 3 to 6 inches will be made. Then , the tissue around the opening within the abdomen wall are stretched and stapled or sutured shut.

Prior to the invention of surgical mesh, it was the only repair procedure for hernias that was available. It's been in use for over a hundred years. It is most likely the hernia repair procedure of your grandfather.

This could be the only solution for patients suffering from massive hernias or who are concerned about possible adverse effects of surgical mesh.

Important points:
- Proven and tried procedure
- Larger incision(s)
It is painful
The recovery period can be as long as up to
Recurrence rates are higher as compared to alternatives to surgery (meaning that you're more likely suffer another hernia)
I would advise against taking this kind of procedure If the recommendation is given by a doctor who is not certified to perform laparoscopic surgeries, that requires additional education. Be sure that he's not leading you to the type of procedure that is right for him and not what's best for you.

Hernia Mesh

A surgical mesh is essentially it is a piece of cloth that is put over the opening in order to seal, strengthen, and secure the herniated part. It is much simpler as opposed to the previous method of stretching the sides and sewing them closed.

The frequency of hernias is also less (nearly not even existent) with mesh , compared to the tension process. The tissue split in the first place due to the tension was just too high to support. Re-tying it and stitching it doesn't do anything to ease the tension. This is the reason why the traditional tension method is so high of recrudivism.

While mesh for hernia repair made of animal (pigs or cattle) is readily available, nearly all mesh used currently is made from synthetic. There are two main reasons long-term durability and price.
Mesh made of animal tissue is degraded over time and becomes weaker. Synthetic mesh, on contrary, is regarded as an indefinite reinforcement for surgical repair.
Another major aspect is the cost. Synthetic mesh can add around 100 dollars to the expense of the process. The biological mesh could increase the cost by as much as $8,000 the price.

There have been many complaints and problems concerning surgery mesh over the years, particularly in the early years of mass use of mesh in hernia repair.

Mesh for the repair of hernias first gained popularity in the early 1990's as laparoscopic surgery for the repair of hernias was recognized as a viable option. Since then the introduction of mesh for surgical repair, advances in technology have made the mesh more secure than ever.

As per the US FDA, "Most of the problems that we have received are related to mesh products that were recalled and are no longer available on sale."

It is important to note however, that there are people who believe that surgical mesh is dangerous. However, I'm not among them. I am a mesh within my body and am thankful for the incredible advancements in technology. I would suggest that you study the subject and then make a choice on your own. It's your body after all.

Laparoscopic Hernia Reconstruction Surgery

Laparoscopic surgery utilizes an electronic "telescope" which is like the flexible scope plumbers uses to view inside the plumbing or the walls. The scope has a light and connects to a viewing monitor to allow the surgeon to observe while performing.

In the course of the procedure, compressed air is introduced in the stomach, causing it to expand and make it explode like balloons. This opens up the space that surgeons need to see and perform the procedure.

Laparoscopic Inguinal Hernia Repair it is common to have three cuts. The largest will be about 1 inch long and located just beneath the navel. It is the place where compressed air and scope get into the abdomen. Two small holes, one lower and one beneath the other, is where the instruments of precision enter, which surgeons use to make repairs (see Figure 3 Figure 3 - Laparoscopic hernia repair diagram).

An actual image of my right-side hernia prior to repair and viewed through the laparoscope exactly as the surgeon sees it, is shown in Figure 4. Laparoscopic Hernia Repair - Before. The lower photo clearly depicts the opening in the tissue that required to be fixed.
the hernia is the same following the repair. It clearly shows how the mesh covers and fills the "hole" within the tissue.

Based on the preferences that your doctor has, after the mesh is placed, it could be held in place using sutures or staples, tacks, the adhesive (glue) or none whatsoever. In the latter the mesh isn't stitched in place. There is no adhesive to secure it in place. It simply sits in position while the gas is able for it to work. When it's in place and the procedure is finished, it is then removed, and it is secured securely in the position.

The application of glue or other substances to secure the mesh together can cause less post-operative discomfort and reduce the risk that staples or tacks could hurt a nerve and create persistent discomfort.

The advantages of Laparoscopic Hernia Repair Surgery

In general, Laparoscopic hernia repair can provide these advantages over open repair procedures:

- Less post-surgery pain

Shorter recovery time

Significantly reduced chance of Recurrence

- Resume work quickly

- Resume regular activities sooner

A surgeon will examine the opposite side for hernias and fix it if necessary.

Incisions are made smaller, which results in smaller scars

Which method is best for You?

My surgeon suggested laparoscopic surgery that included mesh. I am very pleased with the results. Each person's situation is different.

I would suggest that you stay educated (we've provided you with all the information you need) so that you are aware of the recommendations of your surgeon. Trust your surgeon to give you sound guidance. If you aren't at ease with the advice of your surgeon seek out a different one.

How to Select Your Surgeon
In our day and age selecting a surgeon quite similar to selecting an alternative restaurant. Simply search it.

Here's what I did.
I've never been to any primary care physician. Therefore, I googled "internal medicine in my city" (replace my city by yours).
It took a while, but the health benefits are worth it. It was finally a doctor who

received a excellent review after glowing review, and was able to meet me within one week. I attended my appointment and was pleasantly surprised to find the doctor to be as great and as thorough as the reviews claimed.

He suggested me to see my surgeon. His recommendation was now meaningful However, I Googled the surgeon's reviews. After I discovered that he had a good reputation, I was more than willing to work with him.

I strongly suggest this method if don't have a physician or a physician. If you do, it's recommended to still take a look.

It's extremely difficult to alter reviews. Personally, I place more faith on online reviews than the advice of a family member.

I'm hoping this will work very well for you.

Training for Laparoscopic Surgery
Laparoscopic surgery is done with general anesthesia (the kind that can put

you in complete rest). This means that you should not consume food or drink at night after midnight prior to the surgery. A sufficient amount of liquid is required to consume any medication discussed and recommended by your surgeon could be permitted.

Wear loose fitting clothing such as sweatpants to your hospital surgery appointment. Once the surgery is finished and you need to put your pants on again, you'll be grateful that you took the time to dress accordingly. Don't wear an elastic belt.

You'll need ID and credit or debit card to pay for copayment as well as an insurance policy. In addition, you're better off leaving everything other than that at home. All the things you carry can be put in a bag, and then kept in a safe place during your journey. Be aware that if you bring your belongings along, you'll be required to carry it back to your home, even though you might not feel to carry a lot of things.

Due to the general anesthesia , you will be required to let someone else take your home. You will be transported to the vehicle that will pick you up in a wheel chair , by the hospital staff. They will not allow you to take the wheel and drive yourself so plan ahead.

It is ideal to get the prescription for your pain medicine completed prior to procedure, so you don't need to be concerned about filling it once you are back at home. It will be available when you require it.

It is possible to trim the region around your hernia as well as the your groin from the belly button to the bottom of the penis prior to surgery. If not, you can ask a nurse to perform the task for you. Make sure you complete your job properly or the nurse can do the work for you.

Laparoscopic Surgery Recovery
There are many minor side effects from the procedure that you need to take

note of. They are not serious and shouldn't cause much worry.

Constipation after surgery

Constipation can be experienced for between two and five days following surgery. Constipation is an consequence of the general anesthesia as well as any painkillers you are taking. It is normal and shouldn't cause any concern unless it persists for more than five consecutive days.

It is possible to lessen constipation by limiting your opioid pain medication to at night or by not using it in any way. Drinking more fluidly than normal can also assist in reducing constipation.

Pain After Hernia Surgery

Just had surgery. Expect mild to moderate discomfort.

The most likely places of incision are the ones that cause the least amount of pain. Most pain is likely to be felt in the lower abdomen and groin regions.

Your physician may prescribe a painkiller narcotic to help manage the discomfort for a few days. You may also be prescribed Ibuprofen, and/or Tylenol.

If you're allergic to aspirin, do not use Ibuprofen. It is still possible to consume Tylenol (acetaminophen).

Because the half-life for both acetaminophen as well as ibuprofen is brief, it's common to take two of each and then, three hours later take the other. You can alternate between them for three hours rather than waiting six hours to get another dose that is the exact substance. (As always, make sure to consult your physician.)

In my personal experience I was prescribed the painkiller narcotic at night, but only for the first four days. Through the day and until the fifth night, I alternated ibuprofen with Tylenol according to the instructions for approximately one week. I changed to Tylenol exclusively and as advised for another week. After two weeks, I was able to stop any pain medication completely.

Swelling and Bruising

Expect massive swelling and bruising throughout the groin region. The cause of bruising is the blood resulting from the surgery falling down due to gravity. The majority of swelling is actually the result of residual gas left over from the surgery. The swelling should disappear in about 2 weeks it should be totally gone. The swelling should fall within the same time frame and may be a bit faster.

Sore Testicles

Testicular soreness is a short-term consequence. When I say sore imagine sliding into and out of your automobile or chair and just walking around can be like being hit in the groin.

The discomfort will ease gradually as time passes and may last from six to eight weeks, or longer following surgery.

The risk of contracting an infection

As with all surgeries when you undergo a procedure, there is a chance of infections. Check the areas of the incision for any swelling, redness and puss discharge. If you see any symptoms of infection, consult your surgeon at the earliest chance.

Extruding Stitches

After a couple of weeks, I began seeing a rough spot on the uppermost part of the larger cut after it had healed. At first , I thought it was something like a scab. Then, as time passed, it became bigger. It started to feel like an extremely thin and light weight fishing line.

It turns out that it was actually a part of the stitching that was pushing out while the wound was healing.

Six weeks after the surgery, I pulled off the protruding stitch using the help of tweezers, and then removed the stitch.

Returning to Normal Activities

Your surgeon will provide specific details about when you can resume your regular activities. Table 1 provides an example of what to anticipate.

Activity Resumes Following

Shower (No Bathing or Swimming) The following day

Remove Large Bandages Next Day

Remove Smaller Bandages (underneath large) 7 days

Do not lift more than 20 pounds. Two days

Resuming work (No excessive lifting) When you feel able to control the discomfort.

Return to any heavy lifting/strain/exercise 2 weeks

Table 1: Recovery Time for various Activities

My surgeon informed me of an individual patient that had been an MMA fighter who returned to fight in two days. This is a recipe that could be kicked in the butt however, each to his own.

I had surgery on a Friday morning , and was back at work on Monday. However, I work at an office job that requires only a little physical effort. However, I was aching and moving more slowly than I normally do. I also used the elevator to go to one level during the first two days. The third day was the first time I was able to walk up the stairs once more at a moderate speed. At the close of the week, I was able to walk at my usual pace, with only a slight discomfort.

Chapter 8: What Exactly Is Para

Umbilical Hernia?

While they are not restricted to a specific part in the body shenias are named after the places where they can be found, like umbilical, abdominal, etc.

Paraumbilical hernia, which is one of the most common umbilical hernias that adults suffer from occurs in the abdominal wall , above the, below and around but not within the belly button itself (umbilicus).

The abdominal wall is made up of layers of tissue and muscle that reflect each other from left to left. It is situated between the pelvis as well as the thorax. It houses digestive tracts and stomach, and other organs.

What is the cause of a paraumbilical hernia?

Don't be fooled by the hype. Contrary to what many believe that straining or heavy lifting isn't likely to cause a hernia.

Certain medical conditions or activities such as obesity, poor nutrition or smoking can cause increased pressure on the abdominal wall, causing the hernia that is already present to rupture and appear evident.

Umbilical hernias in the abdominal wall occur when fluids (usually that contain fat or intestinal tract) are pushed through a weak part of the 'linea alba' which is the white-line tendon that extends from the rib-cage to the navel.

This tendon connects the right and left sides of muscle to make up the rectus, often known as the six-pack. Hernias develop when a split occurs within the tendon.

The likelihood of a rupture increases when a portion of muscle, tendon or fibrous tissue which forms the abdominal wall becomes weaker. If you cough, strain or sneeze or do anything that increases in pressure within one organ or tissue, that damaged area, ineffective at containing the contents, breaks.

To get a visual idea take a stretch a thin layer of cellophane, resembling the tendon, then create a gap in the middle. When that split or hole is big enough, if it was the linea-alba tendon contents will not be able to remain inside your abdomen. They'd push across from inside to outside (herniate) and create an apparent lump beneath your skin, which could indicate an abdominal hernia.

The symptoms of a paraumbilical hernia
Patients with umbilical hernias have various levels of discomfort. The hernia can initially be apparent when you cause abdominal pressure through breathing, sneezing, or pulling, or standing up to lift weighty objects. However, it is not noticeable when lying down.
This kind of hernia called reducible, can be mildly uncomfortable, but is not necessarily dangerous. In the initial stages the hernia still small, the hernia is usually fat that surrounds the bowel.

They can range in size, from a tiny marble to a much larger.

Many don't complain because they don't exhibit any signs. The hernia is found at the time of a routine medical exam or a check-up. Other patients may experience symptoms like:

O abdominal swelling

Feeling full or bloated

A sharp or dull pain

A persistent abdominal ache

O bumps that show up as you cough.

or swollen bumps disappear

Who is at risk for the Paraumbilical Hernia?

From infants to elderly may develop hernias, most often without explanation. This happened to me. The first time I lived my life and then the next I was living my life with the complication of a Paraumbilical hernia.

Infants

There are some people born with deformities (congenital) that weaken connective tissue in their abdominal-wall muscles. These problems usually heal by the first year of life. However, when they don't heal the hernia could be unnoticed for a long time.

Umbilical hernias that are congenital usually occur shortly after or immediately following birth, and they can heal naturally in the first couple of years.

Infants, especially those that have a premature birth or an unbalanced birth weight and develop umbilical hernias after the umbilical ring isn't able to close. Black newborns are at a greater likelihood of developing a congenital hernia than white infants. If the hernia is not gone away by the age of four it may require surgery to fix the issue.

Hernias are believed to be a result of are inherited. In reality, humans do not inherit hernias however, research suggests that we could have an anatomical weakness in the abdominal muscles, making that area more prone to a hernia forming.

Adults

Repair of abdominal wall and umbilical hernia, is a standard procedure for older adults. Even if there was not any congenital defects as an infant, the occurrences later in life can result in the development of paraumbilical hernias. The risk is higher for older men as are women who are obese, overweight or have had multiple pregnancy.

The Reasons

Below are the actions or medical conditions which may be the cause of sudden increase abdominal pressure until rupture could occur and reveal an abdominal hernia.

Activities

O Crying

Physical exercise

Sneezing that is persistent

O Straining to urinate

A. Traumas to the abdominal area

Affirmation of bowel movements

o Constipation

o smoking (long-term cough)

o A sudden violent cough

o Lifting large objects

Medical Problems

o Obesity

o Diarrhea

o Pregnancy

o Liver disease

o Prior surgery

Cystic fibrosis

o Poor nutrition

o Family family history

A mass or tumor

Prostate cancer that has grown

Un-descended testicles

Obsessed abdominal girth

o Collagen vascular disease

1. Previous open appendectomy

o Abdominal cavity fluid that is excessive

The abdominal wall

Obstructive pulmonary chronic disease

Peritoneal dialysis for treating kidney failure

A swollen abdomen cavity. abdominal cavity

Can an umbilical Hernia be prevented?

Hernias that are born can't be avoided and there's little that you could do to stop parts of your abdominal wall from weakening however the chance to develop one in the future in life can be reduced.

Your aim should be to reduce abdominal pressure. In reducing pressure inside your abdominal wall isn't going to stop the development of a hernia but it can prevent an existing hernia from growing through a weak area.

After you have cleared the procedure with your physician Make a few adjustments to your lifestyle that can increase the odds of avoiding surgery, including:

Make sure you drink plenty of fluids

Maintain an appropriate weight

Make sure you are using the correct methods when lifting.

Don't smoke, it can cause coughing

Exercise to strengthen muscles

Consume high-fiber grains, fruits vegetables, and other fruits

You can also use an stool softener

TREATMENT:

Hernias that are present in adults will not disappear and you can't exercise them away. There is only one way you can fix hernias is to undergo surgery. All other options are temporary.

Umbilical hernia belts , trusses and

I'm not one for the idea of putting a band-aid over it' but using different strokes for different people mean that people could benefit from low-cost belts and clothing specifically designed to put pressure on the hernia to hold it in its place.

These devices, typically used to offer relief from symptoms as a temporary protection, don't have the best performance record and may actually cause the hernia to become more severe.

Belts that are placed around the abdomen's middle is one example. It could cause an increase in abdominal pressure.

In the end, you can't fix your umbilical hernia using external devices that are designed to help keep the hernia in place. Talk to your physician for guidance.

Exercises for Hernia

It isn't possible to do enough sit-ups or crunches to heal hernias, since they don't grow because of weakness in abdominal muscles. Hernias in the umbilical region are caused by weak tissue or muscle known as 'fascia'.

The exercise will build muscle however, it will not heal fascia. Be cautious when exercising prior to consulting with your physician.

I ignored the advice of my doctor and pushed myself too far with the core exercises like sit-ups, crunches and more. These activities raise the pressure in my abdomen which is exactly what you must avoid. They can also aggravate the symptoms of hernia.

Hernia Medication

A single medication will not repair the hernia. In the case of treating an umbilical hernia will only address the discomfort and pain that is caused by the hernia.

What's the danger?

Hernias can be a risk to become "incarcerated" in the event of an increased pressure inside like constant breathing, lifting heavy, or coughing. A portion of your intestine, or abdominal tissue could traverse the ruptured barrier and in the hernia sac and then become trapped or imprisoned, and unable to escape into the cavity.

Incarceration

If abdominal pressure causes stomach content (intestines and the fat) through the hole or defect and to the hernia sac the organs may swell and get trapped or twisting and interfere with the blood supply to the organ.

When an intestine loop or abdominal tissue becomes trapped in an "out" location and is unable to move or be redirected into its own cavity It has been "incarcerated".

An older person will be more at risk than infants and a young child to suffer from incarceration or obstruction of the intestinal tract. Although you should be aware and seek medical attention immediately An incarcerated hernia is not an immediate concern.

The signs of Incarcerated Hernias

If your hernia ruptures and it ruptures its wall due to pressure inside caused by an incident such as lifting weights or coughing and you feel an intense pain that will not disappear. Other signs of incarceration include:

o nausea

o excessive pain

o excessive swelling

o excessive vomiting

o excessive constipation

The bulge may be discolored

It is impossible to push back into position

Strangulation

After being imprisoned, the risk of strangulation is increased. If this happens an organ or tissue protruding through the damaged tendon or muscle is deficient in blood supply. Strangulation blocks circulation outside the twisted area completely.

If surgery is not performed urgently to relieve strangulation tissues that extend beyond the twisted area is likely to become infected (gangrene) as well as die due to the absence in blood circulation.

The infection may spread throughout the abdominal cavity, putting you in a dangerous situation. It is clear that your organ is in danger of dying. You should consult a doctor immediately!

The signs of strangulation

The constriction or compression of the organ may result in severe irritation and damage to the tissues which indicates that blood and oxygen flow to your intestine has been reduced. The skin around the area will change to an intense purple or red color. it could be accompanied by

O fever

o nausea

o diarrhea

o vomiting

o severe pain

o pale complexion

O weakness or dizziness

A tenderness or tingling in the region

A stomach swelling or constipation

A hernia that is strangulated is a medical surgical emergency. Consult your physician or go to an emergency.

Consultation with the doctor

During your exam the doctor will inquire about your medical history. They may also be able to identify your hernia using a visual physical examination. If the hernia appears to be less during the exam, it could require an imaging test , such as Ultrasound or CT scan to determine the condition.

Questions your Doctor may ask

Q. Have you vomited?

Q. What's your pain level? 1-10?

Q. What are your symptoms?

Q. How long have you been suffering from symptoms?

Q. Are the symptoms getting worse?

Q. Do you suffer from a persistent cough?

Q. Are you gaining weight lately?

Q. Have you undergone surgery in this region?

Q. Did you experience any trauma to the region?

Q. Does anyone in your family have an hernia?

Q. Do you perform heavy lifting or strain?

Questions to ask your doctor

Q. What type of hernia would i have?

Q. What are the recommended treatments?

Q. Are there any other options for me?

Q. What is my chance of complications?

Q. Do you suggest an expert?

Q. Do I have to expect my symptoms to improve?

Q. What are the signs of an emergency?

Q. Can I continue exercising?

Diagnose of an Umbilical Hernia

Healthcare specialists have access to cutting-edge equipment, but a physical exam could be all you need to establish if you're suffering from an abdominal hernia. The diagnosis begins by asking you questions to obtain your complete medical background. They also perform a visual exam.

Visual Exam

One of the first things they check for is a swelling within the navel area or close to it. A swollen or enlarged umbilical hernia is apparent to an untrained eye. making the diagnosis.

If the hernia isn't evident, you could be required to sit bent over, sit down, cough or any of these actions to increase the pressure inside your abdomen, causing the hernia, in case you already have one, to expand. If you cough for example the area affected may develop an indentation.

Physical Exam

A medical professional will check the area affected for the presence of bulges when pressure in your body is increased due to coughing, for example. If the physical and visual tests aren't able to provide the diagnosis, either an ultrasound scan or CT scan might be required.

Ultrasound

Ultrasound (sonography) makes use of the technology of sound waves to create images of the inside of your body . It shows its results to a monitor for the technician to interpret.

A typical example is when a woman who is pregnant is subjected to ultrasound tests where the ultrasound technician or radiologists apply an oil-based gel on her abdomen, then rubs an ultrasound transducer over the gel and displays images of her baby on a monitor.

The data is transmitted to a computer monitor that is recorded and reviewed by a radiology specialist who analyzes the images and then either discuss the results with you or provide an update to the doctor who arranged your exam.

CT Scan (Computerized Tomography)

If a physical or a visual examination fails to yield an clear conclusion, your physician might recommend an CT scan to confirm the diagnosis that is correct.

A CT scan gives more in-depth information than just one X-ray. The technology can be utilized to identify a hernia combing several X-ray images of your abdomen taken from various perspectives, then using computer-generated processing to produce an image of a cross-section of these images of soft tissue.

What are they looking for?

A problem or obstruction that could be causing discomfort, swelling, nausea vomiting, fever, or pain.
Doctor's diagnosis
Your doctor might or may not require X-rays, or a CT scan of your bowel. However after your exam, a consulting with a surgeon could be suggested. Don't be fooled, this is a normal procedure. the only way to fix hernias at this point is by surgery.

The Surgeon should be consulted.

During the exam, be prepared to answer the questions the surgeon may ask you to gauge your capacity to endure surgery. After the exam , you will consider options for treating the hernia you have identified.
The Doctor may ask questions
Q. Have you vomited?
Q. What is your level of pain, 1-10?
Q. What are your symptoms?

Q. How long have been you experiencing symptoms?

Q. What caused you to notice the symptoms?

Q. Are the symptoms worse or better?

Q. Do you suffer from a persistent cough?

Q. Did you gain weight recently?

Q. Have you undergone surgery in this region?

Q. Have you experienced any trauma?

Q. Do any of your family members have a hernia?

Q. Do you perform any lifting or straining take place?

Q. Would you like for surgery?

After the examination If it's the opinion of your surgeon that you're a suitable candidate, surgery could be suggested without additional visit.

Questions you can ask your surgeon

Q. How long have you been repairing hernias?

Q. How many hernias have been fixed?

What type of surgery would you rather have?

Q. Open vs. laparoscopic?

Q. What is the downside to either?

Q. Which of the following has a lower recovery?

Q. How do you calculate your frequency rate?

Q. Mesh vs. Sutures?

Q. How does the mesh get attached?

Q. Can a mesh implant detach?

Q. What kind of anesthesia is administered?

What is my chance of complications?

Q. Do I want to have visible marks?

Q. Do you know if your patients have had any issues?

Q. Should I be expecting chronic pain?

Q. What are the best ways to treat chronic pain?

When should I be able to return?

Q. What can I do to speed up healing?

Q. When can I start exercise?

Pre-surgery preparation

The instructions will include:

The date on which when your surgery will be scheduled

What time should you show up at admissions

Outpatients must have designated drivers

If You Smoke,

You should cut back as far as you are able to

You should avoid smoking the day prior to surgery

You should definitely not smoke on the day before surgery.

Surgery Day

No drinking or eating after 12am.

A shower with antibacterial soap

Wear clothing that is loose and comfortable. clothes

You can take the medication by taking an intake of water

o do not take diabetic medication

o bring your asthma inhaler

o bring your contact lenses case

Do Not Wear

o lipstick, mascara, nail polish, make-up

Jewelry like watches, earrings, watches or bracelets

Don't Bring

Checkbook, credit cards as well as cash or valuables

Surgery Day

Nurses will prepare you by asking questions and performing vitals and shaving your abdomen and connecting monitors.

When you're prepared and ready for surgery The surgeon and anesthetist will meet with you to make sure that you are mentally and physically ready for surgery.

Following the consultation, you'll be transferred to an operating room, where you will be administered an Anesthesia. From that point on, you'll be completely memoryless.

Your surgeon may not be able to determine the dimensions of the hernia prior surgery because of fat that has been stuck in the sac of hernia. After the incision has been made and it is then the "hernia sac" is separated. The surgeon then replaces the hernia sac back to its normal position and applies sutures when the hole in the muscle isn't too big. If the wound is more extensive the surgeon can insert mesh over it to seal and cover the wound. Mesh implants or sutures will remain in place for a long time.

Mesh Implant

If the defect is greater than (2cm) suturing may not be the most effective option to fix the hole in the muscle.

Once that has been determined an appropriate mesh covering will be positioned over the opening and stitched or stapled to the area. After the mesh is secure and the opening inside the muscle has been sealed, the opening is sealed.

Open vs. Laparoscopic Surgery

A minor paraumbilical hernia may be treated with surgery or a procedure however using the surgery known as laparoscopic (minimally invasive) procedure isn't appropriate to all people. Patients who are overweight or have undergone abdominal surgery, or suffer from medical issues that are complex, could require open surgery.

Open Surgery
Mesh isn't used to treat small hernias, with very low recurrence. In the (original) procedure the surgeon creates one incision which provides an unobstructed view and is large enough to allow for the insertion of instruments. Once the wound is healed by sutures, they are then used to seal the incision.
Surgery Open Surgery Benefits
Increases visibility into the rupture
It helps secure sutures or mesh
There is a lower chance of damaging other organs

Are not discouraged by the appearance of old scar tissue

Disadvantages of Open Surgery

The procedure can be an invasive procedure

A cut will be huge and noticeable

The risk of bowel cancer or the risk of vascular damage

Laparoscopic Surgery

Surgery that is open is not uncommon and will always be a necessity however, the trend is towards minimally surgically invasive, leading to a decrease in the frequency of recurrences.

The 1980s witnessed an increase in use of mesh and a shift toward mesh-based hernia surgeries. If the size of your hernia is greater than 3/4 inches (2cm) and your surgeon is able to determine that mesh is needed, a laparoscopy can be done.

Instruments for medical use are inserted through tiny cuts in the abdomen after the abdomen has been covered with carbon dioxide gas as well as a high definition camera (laparoscope) is put inside one of the incisions.

The gas permits the camera to send an image that is clear to a nearby monitor which gives surgeons a full view of the abdomen during the procedure. Other instruments are employed to remove this herniated area from the abdominal wall, then return the sac to its normal location and then secure the mesh into the correct position using staples, sutures or staples.

The laparoscopic procedure however, isn't suitable for all patients. If you've had an abdominal procedure in the past, or are overweight, an open procedure might be needed.

Laparoscopic Benefits

Incisions made in the skin will be very small but noticeable

A reduced the risk of bowel or injuries to the vascular system

A lesser loss of blood

There is less pain after surgery

A lesser requirement for pain medications
There is a lower chance of getting ill
o shorter hospital stay
A quicker recovery time after surgery
Laparoscopic Advantages and Disadvantages
It's more intrusive
O is a risk of close to organ injury
It is difficult to place the mesh
o movement problems.
o postoperative bowel obstruction
Discuss with your healthcare professional on the advantages and disadvantages of laparoscopic in comparison to. sutures and open. mesh. My surgeon's method included open and laparoscopy in order to insert mesh implants.

After Surgery

After your outpatient or inpatient umbilical hernia repair, your will be transported to recover and monitored for any signs of bleeding, shock, or infections until fully stabilized and discharged. You should expect to stay in recovery for 2 hours, perhaps longer.

Discharge

If the hernia in your umbilical cord is treated in an outpatient manner and you are discharged the same day, unless there was a problem after surgery that caused the need to admit you to a hospital for additional treatment.

Once you have stabilized After stabilization, your surgical or nursing staff will guide the patient on how look after the incision, and give you contact numbers to dial if you encounter problems or have queries.

To ensure your safety

You will need to drive back to your home

o do not operate machinery

You can have someone around you at all times

If you do not satisfy these requirements the healthcare professional may, be hesitant to admit you to be observed.

Complications of surgery

Every surgical procedure has potential for complications. The complications that are not blood clots are usually detected before you are allowed to go home.

Chronic Pain

Studies show that 20 percent of patients who have hernia meshes will experience chronic pain. If you go through minimally invasive laparoscopy (said to reduce pain after surgery) as well as open surgical procedures, as soon as your first day, you're likely to be hurting.

Because of anesthesia, pain will be reduced in the course of your recovery However, before you are released , you will be given medications to ease the pain.

Partially Collapsed Lung

You might find it difficult to breathe deep enough to take in the air. Post-operative pain, which is common following surgery, makes us take short breaths, which can contribute to partial collapse of the lungs.

Blood Clots

If you're overweight or inactive, and particularly if you smoke, you're more likely to develop blood clots, in which the blood thickens and forms semi-solid masses. Typically, they are found on the feet, blood clots could develop anywhere in your body.

The main risk associated with blood clots is that they may be formed after discharge and could spread to other parts of your body like the lungs.

Be alert for any unusual swelling in the site. If you notice a breathing problems or chest pain following the procedure, it could be a sign that a clot has moved.

This problem requires immediate attentionas it could cause a sudden blockage in one of the major blood vessels in the lung (pulmonary embolism).

Constipation

One of the most common side effects of pain medications is constipation, which is a physical condition that affects the bowels, when we experience:

O hardened, dry stool

o difficulty passing stool

o infrequent, painful bowel movements

To prevent constipation, remain completely hydrated with plenty of fluids. You'll receive an ointment for stool that is prescribed or you can purchase one from your local pharmacy.

Anesthesia Causes Confusing - - Fatigue

If you've heard horror stories of experiencing acute pain or even waking awake during a procedure (rare) it's the job of anesthesia to ensure it doesn't occur. Anesthesia is administered to prevent the patient from having any recall of the procedure, and also to reduce the discomfort.

The patient will awake after surgery feeling a little dizzy or groggy, but once the anesthesia begins to fade, you will be able to get back up. There are other negative effects like a nausea, sore throat or sleepiness.

For those first few days, stay away from operating machines, driving or making major decisions, using alcohol or self-medicating.

If you're older then you could experience fatigue which is a frequent side-effect to last for a few weeks. It is important to be watched to look for any signs of confusion and so on. over the course of several days following surgery, even though the symptoms may last for several weeks or even for months.

Even if you're a highly energetic person, do not 'plow ahead' in an effort to speed up recovery once you've been released. Resuming your regular routine may not be the best choice for you. Give yourself up to 4-6 weeks for adjustment and heal.

Infection

There is no way of getting rid of an infection following surgery. There are instances of infection that can occur however, according to the CDC post-surgery infection rates are extremely rare and less than 2 percent of patients developing even a small infection that occurs around the area of the incision. When you're allowed to return home, ensure that the people that you touch are clean.

Muscle Atrophy

Make sure you move your body. A prolonged period of bed rest or sitting for long periods coupled with little or no exercise, are the fast track to rapid loss of muscle. Following abdominal surgery, be wary however, get up and put your muscles into action.

It's not necessary to go to the fitness studio. Just get busy. In fact, do not lift more than 15 pounds (less than that is recommended) for two weeks after laparoscopic surgery. If you've had open surgery because of the extent of incision, allow at minimum six weeks for healing.

If your surgeon believes that therapy could be beneficial Physical therapists will be suggested to help return to the basics.

Scar Tissue

If you undergo surgery, you'll be left with a mark. It could be large, or maybe it will be small, but when the skin is cut and damaged to the initial layer, it regenerates itself.

Scar tissue can expand, which causes the fabric patch to shrink, pulling off from the defects. It can also be in contact with a bowel and cause constant discomfort. When the mesh no longer can cover the hole the hernia can recur.

Mesh Complications

O mesh movement tugging on or balling
o foreign-body rejection

Some people are allergic to certain substances, which is why their bodies reject them

A Mesh infection (less than 1 %)

If it's defective The recommended remedy is to perform surgery to remove the mesh.

RECOVERY

Nobody will have the exact same experience. Recovery time varies based on a variety of factors, such as what surgery you choose to undergo as well as how extensive your procedure is and your age, physical condition as well as your mental health and more.

Take it easy

In the beginning, I tried to accomplish too much, too quickly however my heart told me "cut it out now!"

If you're like me and are used to a routine filled with strenuous physical activity you might have to cut the pace for a few weeks. I read a few reports that said that in two to four weeks, I would be back to my normal. However, it took me about 6 weeks before my eyes were not at my mid-section 24/7.

It's not unusual to feel pain at the region of the incision, along the abdominal wall, as well as muscle soreness that you'd not thought about. After recovering from surgery you'll be compensating with other muscles, for instance your arms, which you use to lift furniture up and other objects, as opposed to. your legs, abdominals and legs, etc.

It is normal to feel some discomfort in your abdomen area However, if the pain is extreme, consult your physician or visit an emergency room immediately.

Following Surgery Follow-Up

In your next visit, the surgeon will check your incisions, and ask questions to ensure that your progress is in line with the schedule and decide if you'll need to undergo additional surgery.

If you're progressing in the right direction and don't have any complications, you likely will not require another procedure. The surgeon will determine if it is necessary you should schedule another follow-up.

RECUPERATION

Don't be rushed Be yourself, be who you are. You've been through emotional and physical trauma. Take care of yourself just like you would someone you loved.

Allow yourself to heal, but do it according to your pace.

No one is more aware than you of what you're feeling and how you're recovering. Go to the max Then, relax, take a break , and then relax. Your body will inform you that you're done.

Estimated Time to Recover from Umbilical Hernia:

o drive your car 1-2 days

o socialize after 1- 2 weeks

You can walk or jog for a couple of weeks

Strength training after 4 to 6 weeks

Do sit-ups or crunches following 4 to 6 weeks

o perform normal activities 4 - 6 weeks

Full recovery in 8 weeks

Prognosis

The risk of having an occurrence of a hernia in the future is low.

O with laparoscopy, reoccurrence of the procedure is very low

O with open, recurrence could be more frequent

The world should return to normal within a short time
o enjoy!

Umbilical Hernia Facts from the USA
Umbilical Hernia
O is not a genetic trait
The condition can occur at any time
O will be developed within 10% of the population
O is seen in men and women
o common in male infants
It is present in 20 percent of infants
It is common among pregnant women
O is normal in patients with abdominal fluid
O in those who've experienced multiple births
It is common among people who have weak abdominals
It is a common occurrence in patients with liver disease
It is more prevalent in African Americans
O is among the top 10 surgery for outpatients

More than 1,000,000 are repaired annually

About 60% of patients are between 25 and 64 years old

MY PERSONAL EXPERIENCE AFTER-SURGERY

The first week of the year:

o Extremely sore central area

It's hard to get up

I could only lie on my back

o Core pain when having to get out of chair or bed

Use legs and arms to compensate

o Slow and bent over when walking

o Constipated

Second week:

o Less sore core

o A painful core when even getting out of bed

o Core pain when being able to get up from the chair

o Use your legs and arms to compensate

O Holding my breath for a long time

• Not constipated at all

Easily winded

Third week:

O A slight sore center

It's not as slow to move around

The patient was not bent initially however, later

It's not that difficult to get up from your chair or bed

o Use your legs and arms to compensate

Frustrated by slow recovery

A feeling of bloatedness after eating

o Constipated

Fourth week:

Not slow-moving

It's not difficult to stand up

o Not as painful core

o Use legs and arms to compensate

A little bent if standing after sitting

A feeling of bloatedness after eating

o Move well

21-Day Real-Time Record

Week 1

Day 1: Extremely painful in the core. It is difficult to get up from mattress. Utilizing arms to help. Slow movement and bent while walking around the home. I took a pain medication at 4 times a day for 12 hours. (3 in total) I stayed in bed the entire day, reading or sleeping. I was not in the mood to watch TV.

Day 2: Extremely painful in the core. It is difficult to get up from mattress. Slow movement, bent over while walking around the your home. Constipated. There was no pain medication starting today. (I decided to stop taking the pain medication after the second day since they caused constipation.)

Day 3: Sore core area. It's difficult to get up and sit up. Make use of legs and arms to make up for it. Slowly moving, bent over while walking around the your house. Constipated.

Day 4: Not as sore in the in the core area. It's not as difficult to get up and out of the chair. Utilizing your legs and arms to help. Slowly moving, bent while walking around the houses. Constipated.

Day 5: A little more discomfort today in the core. It's not as difficult getting out of bed and into a chair. By using legs and arms to help. Not as slow , not as bent while walking. Easy to tired. Constipated. Car was driven today.

Day 6, Sore in the middle. I was too busy yesterday. It was not as difficult to get up from bed and into a chair. By using legs and arms to make up for the lack of legs. It's not as slow and not as bent while walking. Easy to get winded. The constipation is not a problem.

Day 7: A bit sore on the back of the head. It's not as difficult to get up from the bed and chair. By using legs and arms to make up for the lack of legs. Not as slow and not as bent over. It is easy to get winded. I find myself snoring often.

Week 2

Day 8: A little sore in the core. It is easier to climb up or down using legs and arms to help. The speed is not quite as fast, and not bent at first however, it will be later. Breathing frequently. Constipated.

Day 9: A little sore in the core. It was easy to get out of the chair and bed, using legs and arms to make up for the pain. It's not as slow. Still bent over. Breathing often. Constipated.

Day 10: A little sore in the core. It's not difficult to get up from bed and sit up. Utilizing legs and arms to help. It's not as slow or bent over. I'm holding my breath. I am frustrated that it takes longer to heal. Constipated.

Day 11: A little sore on the back of the neck. It's not too difficult to stand up. With legs and arms, you can make up for. Moving slowly, but not as bent as I would be. I'm not as breathy. It is frustrating that it takes longer to recover. Constipated.

Day 12: A little painful in the core. It's not difficult to get up. By using legs and arms to make up for. Moving slowly, but without bending over. I'm breathing less. It is frustrating that it takes longer to recover. No constipation.

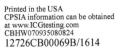

Printed in the USA
CPSIA information can be obtained
at www.ICGtesting.com
CBHW070935080824
12726CB00069B/1614

9 781774 858691